Healing With Yoga
The BRCA Gene and Me

Sarah Brown

Copyright © 2018 Sarah Brown

All rights reserved, including the right to reproduce this book, or portions thereof in any form. No part of this text may be reproduced, transmitted, downloaded, decompiled, reverse engineered, or stored, in any form or introduced into any information storage and retrieval system, in any form or by any means, whether electronic or mechanical without the express written permission of the author.

The views expressed in this work are solely those of the author and do not necessarily reflect the views of the publisher, and the publisher hereby disclaims any responsibility for them.

ISBN: 978-0-244-38701-3

PublishNation
www.publishnation.co.uk

Please seek medical advice before beginning any exercise programme.

Front cover photo: on location at Pigeon Point, Tobago.

Acknowledgements

Firstly, thanks to the consultants, doctors and nurses who took such great care of me during my operations and hospital appointments. The NHS is a precious institution that we should protect at all costs.

I would also like to thank my parents for their unwavering support, love and guidance throughout this process. You are always there for me but never intrusive. I now realise that is a rare gift.

Thank you, Steven, for supporting me throughout. You've been with me during the hardest part of my life. To quote Marilyn Monroe 'If you can't handle me at my worst, then you sure as hell don't deserve me at my best'. Steven, you've definitely seen me at my worst and stayed with me anyway. Thanks for all the cuddles and for putting up with the blood, sweat and tears. Love you always.

Last but not least, big thanks to my beautiful cat Truffles. Thanks for all the licks and purrs.

Thanks to my Mum for editing this book, Steven for the photos and my Dad for being my rock.

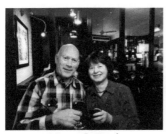 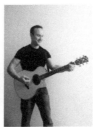 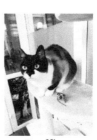

Mum & Dad   *Steven*   *Truffles*

Acknowledgements

Firstly, thanks to the consultants, doctors and nurses who took such great care of me during my operations and hospital appointments. The NHS is a precious institution that we should protect at all costs.

I would also like to thank my parents for their unwavering support, love and guidance throughout this process. You are always there for me but never intrusive; I now realise that is a rare gift.

Thank you, Steven, for supporting me throughout. You've been with me during the hardest part of my life. To quote Marilyn Monroe "If you can't handle me at my worst, then you sure as hell don't deserve me at my best." Steven, you've definitely seen me at my worst and stayed with me anyway. Thanks for all the cuddles and for putting up with the blood, sweat and tears. Love you always.

Last but not least, big thanks to my beautiful cat Truffles. Thanks for all the licks and purrs.

Thanks to my Mum for editing this book, Steven for the photos and my Dad for being my rock.

Mum & Dad   Steven   Truffles

Dedication

For my grandmother Frances who I didn't get the chance to meet and my Auntie Rosalind who didn't get to see me grow up. I dedicate this book to you both. I wish you would have had the same choices as me.

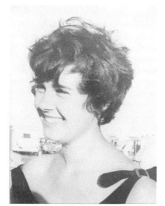

Auntie Rosalind

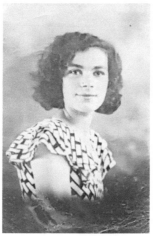

Grandma Frances

Healing With Yoga: The BRCA Gene and Me

Each chapter contains a breathing exercise, yoga posture and a meditation. They can be used alone or combined for a longer sequence.

Contents

Chapter 1: Intuition   1

Yoga to increase intuition   5

- Child's Pose
- Intuitive Breath
- Candle Meditation

Chapter 2: Denial   7

Yoga to shift your perspective   10

- Legs Up The Wall
- Breath Counting
- Words Matter

Chapter 3: Stress   12

Yoga for Stress   16

- Forward Fold
- Alternate Nostril Breathing
- Mantra

Chapter 4: Towards Surgery   18

Yoga for fear   22

- Side Stretch
- Cooling Breath
- Heart Breath

Chapter 5: Being Sure   24

Yoga for releasing tummy tension   27

- Tummy Relaxer
- Hold & Release
- Belly Breath

Chapter 6: Bye Bye Boobies   29

Yoga for releasing emotional tension   32

- Cat/Cow Stretch
- Lion's Breath
- Healing Light

Chapter 7: The Great Nipple Debate   34

Yoga to energise   38

- Cobra Pose
- Breath Of Fire
- Recharge

Chapter 8: Analyse Me   40

Yoga for clear thinking   44

- Standing Position & Half Sun Salutations
- Mind Cleanse
- Walking Meditation

Chapter 9: Getting the Date   47

Yoga for anxiety   50

- Downward Facing Dog
- Bumblebee Breath
- Picture Perfect

Chapter 10: Preparation   52

Yoga to prepare for surgery   55

- Warrior 1
- Peaceful Breath
- Shower Meditation

Chapter 11: Recovery   57

Yoga to aid recovery   63

- Seated Butterfly
- Muscle Tense and Release
- Affirmation

Chapter 12: One Down, One To Go   65

Yoga for increasing determination   69

- Warrior 2
- Let Go
- Music Therapy

Chapter 13: Staying Calm — 71

Yoga for calming the mind — 76

- Bridge Pose
- 4-7-8 Breathing
- Calming Scents

Chapter 14: Waking Up — 78

Yoga for panic — 81

- Neck Release
- Coloured Breath
- Body Scan

Chapter 15: The Long Night — 83

Yoga for survival — 88

- Post Op Exercises
- Magic Hands
- Walking Meditation (see Chapter 8)

Chapter 16: Heal Thy Self — 90

Yoga to aid healing — 93

- Supine Butterfly
- Peaceful Breath
- Mind Power

Chapter 17: Beginning To Heal　　　　　　95

Yoga to support healing　　　　　　　　　99

- Lay Over Blanket
- Mindful Breath
- Crystal Healing

Chapter 18: Getting Stronger　　　　　　101

Yoga to build strength　　　　　　　　　105

- Lunge
- Three Part Breath
- Taste Meditation

Chapter 19: Bad News　　　　　　　　　107

Yoga for coping with bad news　　　　　　111

- Tree
- Triangle Breath
- Here and Now

Chapter 20: Staying Positive　　　　　　113

Yoga for a positive mind　　　　　　　　116

- Supine Twist
- Riding The Waves
- Gratitude

Chapter 21: Dark Days   **118**

Yoga to aid sleep   123

- Supine Pigeon
- Sleepy Breath
- Sweet Dreams Meditation

Chapter 22: New Beginnings   **125**

Yoga for acceptance   131

- Smoke and Light
- Standing Twist
- Thought Awareness

Chapter 23: My Own Yoga Studio   **133**

Yoga for letting go   137

- Twisted Lunge
- Dandelion Breath
- Loving Kindness Meditation

Chapter 24: Rock Bottom   **140**

Yoga for anger   145

- Wide Legged Forward Fold
- Finger Breathing
- A Gift From Anger

Chapter 25: Looking Ahead   **147**

About Sarah   **152**

Chapter 1: Intuition

'Satya' is one of my favourite words. It means 'truth' in Sanskrit, an ancient Indian language.

This is my truth.

I've fallen apart, changed and healed again and again.

I want to share my story and how the magic of yoga has helped me.

In November 2014 I had a blood test which would change my life.

A few months previously my Dad found out he had both the BRCA 1 & 2 gene mutations. I decided to find out if they had been passed on to me.

If I had one or both genes it would mean that I would have an 87% risk of getting breast cancer and a 50-60% risk of getting ovarian cancer. Compared to the general population of women, who have an 11% risk of breast cancer and a 1.5% risk of getting ovarian cancer, this is very high.

My Dad had been encouraged to have the test by his first cousin who at the time had breast cancer. She didn't have the strength to get tested so she asked my Dad to take it. Then we could find out if it was in our family.

My Dad (touch wood) is the fittest and healthiest man I know. He was sixty-eight when he was tested and still taught fitness classes. I didn't consider for one moment there could possibly be anything wrong with him.

I was completely devastated when I found out that he had both mutated genes – something happening to my Dad is my worst nightmare. However, when we researched, we found out the gene in men isn't nearly as serious. It would mean him having regular blood tests to screen for prostate cancer and he should probably have some form of breast screening too.

Once I knew my Dad had the mutated gene, my first reaction was not to have the genetic test. I didn't want to know. Why would I want to know? I didn't want to live my life knowing that I was more than likely to develop cancer.

Around this time, I met my boyfriend Steven. An intense relationship from the start, this seemed to take up a lot of my emotional energy and it took my mind away from the gene. I did tell him a condensed version about the gene, but I skimmed over the facts with upbeat positivity.

Even though my gut reaction was not to have the test, all the facts and figures played on my mind. Unless I had the test, I would wonder forever. I was almost sure I didn't want children but if I did have them then potentially I could pass on the mutated gene unknowingly.

I am a yoga teacher and fairly hippy in my thinking (at least that's how my boyfriend would describe me!). On one hand I thought that even if I did have this problem I would be okay as I lived a healthy lifestyle and surely this would make a difference.

I also rightly or wrongly believed that the universe would steer me in the right direction. So I listened. And listened. I looked for signs and clues. But nothing came. Instead I looked within to my intuition. What was my gut telling me to do? It turns out my gut told me to take the test.

So here I am in this hospital room with my Dad and the most insincere genetic counsellor I have ever seen (and I've met a few). Nobody can have a genetic test without first having counselling. A good idea in theory but you need to see the right person.

She presented me with the cancer statistics and told me that if I had the gene I would definitely have to undergo risk reducing surgery. This would mean losing my breasts and ovaries. As if that wasn't upsetting enough she then asked me if I was angry with my Dad for possibly passing on a mutated gene to me! I could never feel this way, as obviously, it's completely not his fault.

After this ordeal I was given the blood test and told I would have to wait 4 weeks for the result. It was going to be a long wait.

I remember leaving the hospital with my Dad, seeing the strain and stress etched on his face. I hoped that I didn't have the faulty gene. Obviously, I didn't want it for me but more than anything else I was worried about my Dad. His Mum had died of ovarian cancer shortly before I was born and his sister died of breast cancer at the age of 45. I didn't want him to see me face the same fate.

Dad and I were silent for a while, trying to let everything sink in, but then in his typical style he said, 'Let's get a drink'.

We went for a lovely meal and shared a bottle of wine. We laughed a lot and did silly impressions of the counsellor. That's the thing about my Dad...he always knows how to make every situation better. His wit and humour can diffuse even the most difficult occasions.

During the long wait for the result I was busy with work. As well as teaching yoga, I was the studio manager at a large yoga studio, 'Studio 666'. I was also travelling a lot. Steven lives in Leeds and I am in London and every week I went up to spend three days with him.

By now it was coming up to Christmas and I had my work night out. I was really looking forward to letting my hair down and I'd even brought a new outfit. I got ready at my friend's house and enjoyed being pampered as she did my make-up. I felt good. I looked good. I had a great night. What could go wrong?

The next day the letter from the hospital arrived. It looked so innocent hiding in its small white envelope but the sight of it made my head spin. I took some deep breaths to steady myself before I opened it.

I had BRCA 1.

Yoga To Increase Your Intuition

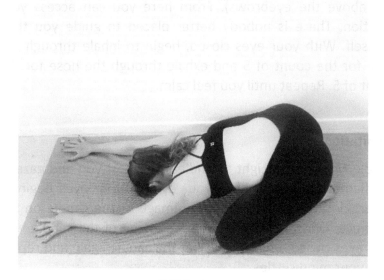

Child's Pose

Pose:

Child's Pose: In kneeling position, make your knees the distance of your mat and bring your toes together. Now press your bottom towards your heels and reach your arms forward along the mat. Gently move your shoulders away from your ears. Rest your forehead on the mat (use blocks if it cannot reach). Feel the stretch along your spine and breathe deeply. Stay here for 5-10 breaths.

Breath:

Intuitive Breath: Sit comfortably and turn your inner gaze to the third eye (this is the point in the centre of the forehead, just above the eyebrows). From here you can access your intuition. There is nobody better placed to guide you than yourself. With your eyes closed, begin to inhale through the nose for the count of 5 and exhale through the nose for the count of 5. Repeat until you feel calm.

Meditation:

Candle Meditation: Light a candle in front of you and gaze at the flame. Try not to blink your eyes. If your eyes begin to water, close them and focus the image of the candle on the third eye. Once you cannot see the image of the candle with your eyes closed, begin to gaze at the candle again and repeat until your mind settles.

Chapter 2: Denial

I found out the result in the lead up to Christmas 2014. When you find out bad news you go through a cycle of feelings: denial, anger, bargaining, depression and finally acceptance.

I went through all of these and back many times and not necessarily in that order.

My favourite was denial. I spent a lot of time here. This was a great place to be and kept me going for months. During this time, I attended an advanced yoga teacher training. Part of yoga training is to share your thoughts and feelings so you can leave all your emotional baggage at the door and become a better teacher.

I shared and shared in these sessions. I'm a shy person normally but I found comfort being around strangers and really found that I could open-up. My teacher for the course told me that I would be fine as cancer could only survive in an acidic body. Therefore, if I kept my body in an alkaline state then there would be no way that I could contract cancer.

This of course made me feel better. I already led a healthy life. I've always been fit. I work out, swim and have a daily yoga practice. I watch what I eat. I would be absolutely fine. No need for any risk reducing measures. Nothing to worry about.

I then became adamant that as I had an awareness of my body then I would automatically realise if something was wrong. I was extremely sensitive to any changes. I always knew when I was ovulating so surely I would know if I was going to develop cancer?

I'd had breast lump scares before and each time I knew the lump was there without actually feeling it. What I'm saying is that I'm sensitive to my body's changes so this made me feel invincible.

I also believe that everything happens for a reason and all things turn out as they should. I decided that if I was going to get cancer then I was going to live my life to the full until that point.

What followed was in retrospect a very self-destructive period. I completely blocked out thoughts of the gene from my mind and threw myself into work and my new relationship. If I made myself busy enough then I thought that it couldn't catch up with me. As I said denial is a great place to be.

Armed with my new lust for life I had a great time. I went on countless exotic holidays with my boyfriend, theatre trips and days out.

What freaked me out and still does is that I've always had the mutated gene. Since birth. All through school, college, university. Through every job, relationship, good and bad experience it's always been there like a time bomb ticking away. It blew my mind.

I've always had a lot of energy, more than most and I rarely get tired. I also have a thirst for new experiences and I'm forever changing my work and interests. At times, I've found it hard to fit in with others as the way I wanted to live my life seemed so different.

I began to think of the faulty gene as my driving force. It made me special. It was the reason I had such zest for life. Let's face it, if you have impending disaster hanging over your head, then you are going to have the energy and enthusiasm to enjoy every second of every day.

I decided my mutated gene was nothing scary. It was my friend – it fuelled my ambition and urge to learn new things. I'd keep my body healthy and alkaline and I'd be just fine.

Therefore, it just goes to show that the difference between an ordeal and an adventure is quite simply perspective.

Yoga To Shift Your Perspective

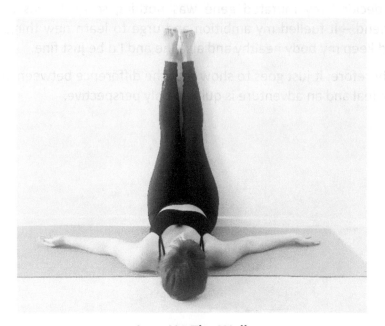

Legs Up The Wall

Pose:

<u>Legs Up The Wall</u>: This is a great way to shift your perspective as you are literally turning your body upside down. In foetal position, manoeuvre against the wall so your bottom touches. Now swing your legs up so they are completely supported by the wall. Your arms can rest by the side of your body, overhead or hands can rest on your belly. Let your legs relax completely. Stay here for at least 5 minutes.

Breath:

Breath Counting: Sit comfortably with a straight spine and relax your shoulders. With your eyes closed begin to count your breaths. Inhale '1', exhale '2', inhale '3', exhale '4' and so on. If you get distracted then begin again. See if you can count to 20.

Meditation:

Words Matter: Take a deep breath and exhale through the mouth. Repeat a few more times. Now choose a word that may help to give you a new perspective. Perhaps it is 'patience'. Perhaps it is 'grace'. For me the word is 'calm'. Any word will do, letting this meditation be as individual as you. Continue to repeat this word as it resonates in your mind and travels through your body. Every time you get distracted, gently bring yourself back to the word that has been within you all along. Now open your eyes and move forward.

Chapter 3: Stress

I was happily in denial and keeping myself busy. Friends and family tried to talk to me about the risks but I blocked them out. I would be okay. Statistics didn't mean a thing to me.

I went to meet a friend one day in town and we had a great day out in the sunshine. I made my way home more than a little tipsy with the feeling of sun on my skin. Sitting on the bus I was about to put my earphones in when I saw her. The lady with a headscarf. The lady with cancer.

She looked so frail, so thin and so very, very sick. I tried not to look at her but I couldn't help it. A ton of bricks hit me all at once that this could be me very soon. I couldn't breathe, I couldn't talk as the realisation sank in. I didn't tell anyone about the lady on the bus but my perspective shifted, my world tilted.

As soon as I got home I researched if I could have any screening. Instead of being a sitting duck maybe I could be screened and at least have some warning that the cancer was coming.

During my initial unhelpful counselling at the genetics clinic they told me the only route would be surgery, but maybe they were wrong. Screening could be the perfect answer. I would be proactive but not undergo surgery.

With the help of my Mum I found out that I could have a regular CA125 blood test and a vaginal scan to check if there was evidence of ovarian cancer. Some reports said this would be a helpful indicator, but most said that as ovarian cancer is so fast growing the test did not save lives. Ovarian cancer is dubbed 'the silent killer' for this reason and also the symptoms are very similar to period pains, i.e. backache, IBS or just bloating.

My parents paid for me to see a specialist consultant in this area. He reviewed my family history (which is bleak reading as cancer is so prevalent) and told me that I would be fine if I was screened as any signs of cancer could be caught early and treated. This was a huge relief and it felt like a weight had been lifted from my shoulders.

For the next 8 months I had regular CA125 blood tests and vaginal scans to check for ovarian cancer. I also had an MRI to check for early signs of breast cancer.

The blood test and scan were fine but the MRI scan made me very sick as they had to inject dye into my body. I also felt very claustrophobic whilst being scanned, but holding Steven's hand throughout helped. All in all, the MRI was unpleasant but I was told I would need it yearly so figured I could put up with it.

I enjoyed the feeling of safety I had from being screened. I felt like I was doing something and action felt good. Everyone in my life seemed to have an opinion but I was happy that I was taking a sensible route. It had been very hard for me at first to tell people about my faulty gene as I am a private person (yes I know I am now writing a book!) but in retrospect this was an important step towards acceptance.

My work colleagues were the most difficult. The ladies in the office at Studio 666 were nosy, pushy and generally unpleasant. They thought nothing of making me feel uncomfortable as they probed me for answers.

Apart from them, my close friends, parents and Steven were extremely supportive. It must have been very hard for them to come to terms with and we all had so many unanswered questions.

I overheard Steven on the phone to his Mum one night. He was telling her that he found it really difficult to be with me. It seemed to him I was living as if it was my last few years. I could see why he thought that. I was spending all my money on having a good time and pushing myself to the limit, over exercising and hardly sleeping. I felt that I didn't want to miss anything. By then I was 37 and the risk of contracting cancer increases when you get closer to 40. Time was running out.

This together with a hectic work schedule and hours of travel ended in me collapsing. Steven and I had been enjoying some early summer sunshine in the park. We'd had a gentle cycle ride, followed by a leisurely stroll, when I suddenly felt uncontrollably dizzy. Before I could say anything, apparently, I fell to the ground and began fitting, violently banging my head.

The next thing I remember is waking up and being very confused. It took me a while to realise where I was and to recognise Steven. He told me afterwards I actually passed out three times but I have no recollection. This is the first time I had ever collapsed. A control freak even in that situation, I put myself into the recovery position! There happened to be a doctor walking past who stopped to help. She said I should go to the hospital to be checked but I refused. So with bruised arms, legs and a grazed face we went home. Steven did all he could to persuade me to go to hospital but I was adamant.

I felt fine the next day and got on the train back to London. During the journey I began to feel dizzy but I did not pass out again. I was however very, very scared. My Mum took me to our local hospital and I was in A&E for 10 hours having tests. After brain scans and heart checks they couldn't find anything wrong with me. They suspected I had epilepsy, so I had to come back for more tests.

In the end, there was nothing wrong with me. They put the collapse down to exhaustion and stress. I didn't even realise I was so stressed, but my body had given me a wake-up call. I needed to start dealing with things better and I needed to look after myself.

Then my Dad's first cousin passed away. Although she had breast cancer it was still a shock as she had been recovering well. Unfortunately, the cancer came back to another part of her body so she faded quickly. She had BRCA 1 & 2 like my Dad. Although she hadn't contracted cancer until she was in her sixties it still played on my mind. It could be me next.

Yoga For Stress

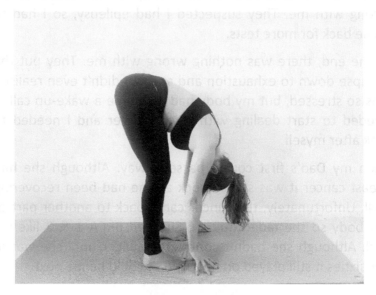

Forward Fold

Pose:

Forward Fold: Stand with your feet hip distance apart and parallel. With a soft bend in your knees, fold forward with a flat back. If your hands cannot touch the floor then use blocks. Bring your weight forward so it is in the balls of your feet. Your legs do not have to be completely straight. Draw your belly up and in. Lift your shoulders away from your ears, soften between your shoulder blades and let your head relax. Inhale through your nose and exhale through your mouth 10 times. Your exhale can be as fierce as you like to relieve stress and tension.

Breath:

Alternate Nostril Breathing: This breathing exercise will calm the mind at stressful times. With your right hand, turn down your index and third finger. Use your thumb to press and close your right nostril. Inhale through the left nostril for 5 counts. Press your ring and little finger to close your left nostril so both nostrils are closed. Hold your breath for 5 counts. Release your thumb, then exhale through the right nostril for the count of 5. Inhale through the right nostril for the count of 5, close the right nostril with your thumb and hold for 5 counts. Then release the ring and little finger then exhale through the left nostril for the count of 5. This is one round. Repeat 5 times.

Meditation:

Mantra: A mantra is a sound or phrase repeated to bring focus and calm to the mind. Find a simple phrase which resonates with you. This is your mantra. I use 'I can cope with anything' or 'I allow life to flow through me'. Sitting comfortably with your eyes closed, repeat your mantra until you believe it. You can use this simple meditation in any situation.

Chapter 4: Towards Surgery

Although I was still being screened I also began to do my own research. My odds weren't good. My aunt died of breast cancer at 45 and my grandmother died of ovarian cancer at 56. I was 37 and the risk increases the closer you get to 40. I was between a rock and a hard place.

I went back and forth between being very, very scared and then a sudden surge of confidence that nothing bad would happen. My gut feeling was that I needed to do something and I needed to do it quickly.

I had no intention of going back to the horrible counsellor at the first genetic clinic, but when I called they assured me I would see another counsellor. This seemed as good place as any to start and I needed information. The information on the computer was confusing and mostly about Angelina Jolie who has the same mutated gene. She had recently had a double mastectomy to decrease her chance of breast cancer.

I'm sorry to say that the second counsellor was not much better than the first. Not quite as patronising, but still very cold. During my time of visiting clinics and hospitals two things are always the same. More often than not I was treated as a number and a piece of meat. Also, although they must have had my records, I had to explain my family history each time I went. Often to the same person again and again and again. On my paternal family tree it's hard to spot those without cancer so it's always a fun discussion!

Anyway, the counsellor told me that my only course of action was to have my ovaries removed and a double mastectomy. If

I didn't do this then I was sure to get cancer and probably die. Another gem about this gene is that the type of cancer you get with the BRCA gene mutation is often the most aggressive type with the worst outcome. It was all good news!

The fall-out from this was huge. I couldn't even contemplate surgery. I couldn't get my head around this option. It just didn't make sense to remove healthy parts of my body 'just in case'. At the back of my mind I was still sure that if I kept up my healthy lifestyle then I would be okay.

The counsellor said the first step would be to remove my ovaries as ovarian cancer is faster growing than breast cancer. She asked if I had children already and I told her that I did not nor did I ever want them. She told me to think really hard about this as there is the option to freeze eggs or embryos that can be used in IVF.

By this point my head was spinning…I had never wanted children – I didn't even like playing with dolls when I was a child. Everyone always said that I would change my mind but at 37 I think you know your own mind. The counsellor urged me told me to talk to my boyfriend.

By then Steven and I had been together for about 6 months. Nobody wants to have 'the baby conversation' that early on in a relationship but I needed to, so I did. Like me he had never wanted children, but his parents wanted him to have a family and were quite disappointed that he didn't have one already. My parents on the other hand had accepted years ago that I wouldn't be breeding.

We talked and talked and talked about freezing eggs or embryos but in the end it didn't feel right for either one of us. We thought it felt like we saying we were interested in having children in the future and we definitely didn't see that happening. I also knew that egg harvesting is very invasive to your body. I was beginning to realise that my body would have to go through a lot anyway.

Once the decision was made I won't lie and say that at times I did not waiver. Thoughts came to me like 'what if Steven changes his mind then he leaves me for someone who could get pregnant', or 'what if I have a change of heart and desperately want children then hate myself for not having the option'. However, I knew that all I could do was trust the feelings we both had at the time. If things changed, they changed. I didn't want to put my body through any extra stress.

Armed with our decision we went to the other side of London to see yet another counsellor at a place with a name that struck the fear of God in me, 'The Menopause Clinic'. I didn't even know that these places existed. But they do. They are often placed right next to the prenatal clinics in hospitals, so they share the same waiting room. When I was sitting there thinking about the fate of my ovaries I was surrounded by babies.

The counsellor at the menopause clinic was downbeat and pointed out that going through the menopause was going to be the most difficult thing ever. As soon as my ovaries were removed I would be plunged overnight into an early menopause and I would have to take HRT. Guess what? HRT increases your risk of getting breast cancer, so you should only go through with it if you are sure about getting your breasts removed too.

Up to this point I thought I might just have my ovaries removed as this would take away most of the risk of getting ovarian cancer and half my chances of getting breast cancer. I then found out this wasn't really an option as I would need to take the HRT to protect my heart and bones.

I knew as much as the next person about the menopause until then, but the counsellor soon pointed out the side effects that I would most probably have (yes she said it was very likely): mood swings, weight gain, hot flushes, night sweats, fatigue, hair loss or thinning and my favourite two – loss of libido and vaginal dryness. There's nothing else that makes you feel like an old woman more than being told you might have vaginal dryness.

The counsellor told Steven that he needed to be very kind and sympathetic to me, then gave me a referral to another hospital to start exploring surgery.

When we left I cried and cried. It was all overwhelming and very real. Steven looked completely shell shocked and I didn't blame him. He was dating an energetic, lively 37 year old who overnight would become menopausal and dried up. I told him that I wouldn't blame him if he wanted to split up with me but he said I was being ridiculous.

On the way home I realised that if I was going to have parts of my body removed then I wanted to be really sure that I definitely had the mutated gene. I wanted to be retested.

Yoga For Fear

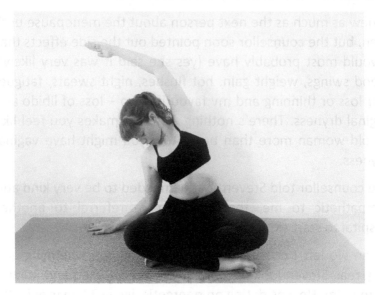

Side Stretch

Pose:

Side Stretch: Sit cross legged or with your legs along the floor. Place your right hand on the floor by the side of your right hip and stretch your left arm overhead. Feel even weight through both sides of your bottom and relax your right shoulder. Enjoy the stretch on your left side as you relax your neck and look towards the floor. Hold for 5 breaths and repeat on the other side.

Breathing:

Cooling Breath: Sit comfortably with a straight back. Fold the sides of your tongue inward. Inhale through your tongue like a straw then close your mouth and exhale through your nose. This will instantly calm you down. Repeat for 2 minutes.

Meditation:

Heart Breath: Lay comfortably on the floor and place your hands on your heart. Begin to breathe deeply into your hands and visualise the colour green. Imagine this colour swirling around your heart and bringing positive energy into your body. Stay here for 2-5 minutes.

Chapter 5: Being Sure

Initially I hoped that I would get retested on the NHS. I explained my worries to my GP and also the first hospital that I visited, but they refused.

I can understand their point of view. I must have seemed crazy as to them the test was fail-safe. From my point of view things can always go wrong. I was thinking of having my ovaries and breasts removed for God's sake, I needed to be sure.

I then went down the route of getting a private test. The company also thought I was mad but were more than happy to take £1,200 for their trouble. The results would take two weeks to come back.

In my heart of hearts I knew the result would be the same, but I obviously hoped it would be different. For a short while it looked like my dreams had come true. After just a week the lab called me to say that there was a difference between the NHS result and their result and they needed to do more tests.

With my hopes raised, I began to believe that I might not have the gene mutation after all. I felt amazing, like the biggest weight ever had been lifted from my shoulders. Unfortunately, the result turned out to be the same. I definitely had the mutated gene. I was crushed.

I received the result when Steven and I had gone to Blackpool for the night. The counsellor called me and broke the news. She gently explained that in her opinion surgery was the only option and it was important that I had it done quickly.

I was devastated and I cried a lot. To have my hopes raised and then dashed was very cruel. Although very understanding, I don't think Steven realised that to me this marked the end of my life as I knew it. Years of visiting hospitals lay ahead and I had to come to terms with losing parts of my body.

At 37 I still felt 18. I looked young for my age and I knew that this would change really quickly. I practice yoga every day, love swimming and working out, but if I had the surgeries my ability to do the things I enjoyed would be limited for a long time.

Despite his reassurance, I was sure that Steven would not want to stay with me. Why would he? I would have no natural breasts and be menopausal. Hardly an attractive thought. Would I even still be a woman? I doubted if I would feel much like one.

The realisation of surgery hit me hard. It was like being struck by lightning. I think the risks of surgery were the scariest for me. If something went wrong during the breast surgery I could actually end up with no breasts. No breasts at all. I wasn't particularly well-endowed, but I wanted to have something.

One good thing to come out of my second test was that the councillor put me in touch with Hospital O for possible ovary surgery. The team in the gynaecology department were a breath of fresh air.

During my first trip, I had blood tests and another vaginal scan. Luckily there were no signs of cancer. I had been really worried in the lead up to the tests. I had started to experience quite severe stomach pains which I feared could be a sign of ovarian cancer. Now I realise it was all stress. My tummy was knotted up with the tension of the situation.

The professor in the department discussed the removal of my ovaries and fallopian tubes. I was asked many times if I wanted to freeze my eggs but my mind was made up. The operation itself seemed straightforward if everything went to plan. Just two small insertions below both hip bones and a small insertion under my belly button. Recovery was around 6 weeks.

The bigger issue was obviously being plunged into an abrupt early menopause. The thought of this scared the hell out of me. Even the thought of taking HRT turned my stomach. It just made me feel old.

I willed myself to get my head around this and I listened carefully all the information. HRT could help suppress some of the symptoms, but it may take a long time to find the right one.

During this first consultation, I signed the forms for the removal of my ovaries and fallopian tubes. I felt like I was signing away my youth. I was placed on the waiting list which was between 3-6 months. As I wasn't deemed urgent the wait could be even longer.

By now I had decided surgery was the only option. If I was going to go down this route I wanted it all done as quickly as possible. 2016 was going to be 'surgery year'. I had lined up this operation with a team that I trusted. I now had to do the same for breast surgery but I didn't have a clue where to start.

Yoga For Releasing Tummy Tension

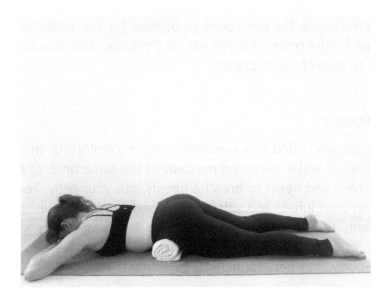

Tummy Relaxer

Pose:

Tummy Relaxer: Place your bolster, pillow or blanket across your mat. Lay over it so that it is just below your belly button. Relax completely for 2-5 minutes. This pose will restrict the flow of blood to the belly so when you carefully come out of the pose, fresh blood will pump through clearing any tension. When coming out of the pose, place your hands underneath your shoulders and push yourself onto your knees.

Breathing:

Hold & Release: Sit comfortably with a straight spine. Inhale and exhale smoothly through your nose then follow this pattern: inhale for the count of 5, hold for the count of 5, exhale for the count of 5. Repeat for 2 minutes and then come back to smooth, even breath.

Meditation:

Belly Breath: I find this meditation more comforting when I place a hot water bottle on my belly at the same time. Lay on your back and begin to breathe deeply into your belly. Feel it rise on your inhale and soften on the exhale. Now envisage a brilliant, bright yellow sunflower which spreads over your belly. Breathe in the scent and feel the warmth move through your body. Stay here for at least 5 minutes.

Chapter 6: Bye Bye Boobies

Ten years previously I had minor breast surgery and I remembered my amazing surgeon. I hoped he would operate on me a second time.

Contacting Mr H was not easy and getting an appointment with him was even harder. Eventually I got my 10 minutes consultation and as I explained my situation, I saw genuine empathy in his eyes.

When you see as many doctors and consultants as I have over the last few years you realise this is rare. I'm not saying that these are bad people, but they are clearly overworked and stressed so maybe the first thing to go in this situation is a bedside manner.

It turned out that Mr H also worked at Hospital B as part of a team of surgeons, consultants and other professionals that helped women in my situation. Up until then I thought I may have to pay for the operation privately, but he assured me that I would get excellent treatment at Hospital B.

Mr H, although sympathetic, is a straight talker. I asked him what he thought I should do. He looked me in the eyes and said, 'If you don't have surgery then you will die of cancer'. Hard to hear but I appreciated his honesty. Deep down I knew he was right.

Mr H examined me and told me that there are two options when it comes to reconstruction after a mastectomy. The first is using fat from the bottom or tummy to reconstruct breasts and the second is using implants. The first option has a more natural look and feel and the second is obviously less invasive.

The words 'double mastectomy' were frightening. On plus side Mr H told me that I didn't have enough fat on me for the first option of reconstruction. I'm a size 8-10 with a few wobbly bits so I was thrilled. It's always nice to feel that you don't have much fat on you!

Actually, I had already decided that I would go for the implant option. I know a few women who've had reconstructions following cancer and they had a lot of trouble with the parts of their body where fat was extracted. One lady couldn't sit down properly for months as when the fat had been taken from her bottom she got an infection which led to complications. Another lady told me that 'she had been butchered' and has dreadful problems with her back after muscle had been taken from there to reconstruct her breasts. No thank you. I wanted the simplest and quickest option.

Mr H explained that he worked with another surgeon on cases like mine. I would need to see Mr J as he would remove the breast tissue during my operation and then Mr H would reconstruct me.

He warned me that my breasts would look very different and I would almost certainly not have any sensation at all. Images of two beaten up melons came to mind. I would just have two things stuck onto my body which wouldn't feel or look like me.

I started to wander if I should have a reconstruction at all. What was the point of having two things stuck on me that I couldn't feel. My nipples have always been very sensitive and I've enjoyed this during sex. The thought of no sensation at all was horrible.

I got home and looked in my wardrobe. I thought about all the clothes that I wouldn't be able to wear again if I didn't have breasts at all or if they changed radically. I wear casual clothes most of the time but I have a number of pretty dresses I wear on nights out and holidays that would look all wrong. If I had no breasts at all what would I be able to wear?

I know there are plenty of women who are flat chested naturally but let me explain about my figure. I'm curvy. I have hips, a bum and shapely legs. This is balanced out by my breasts. If I didn't have these then I would look like a pear.

During this time I also struggled to look at my naked body in the mirror. I know lots of women struggle with this one but although I've never been super confident about my body, I've been happy enough. Now I knew change was imminent I found I didn't want to remember what I looked like now.

Steven always complimented me on my figure. I had to keep reminding him that things were about to change and I didn't know how I would end up. He said it wouldn't make any difference to him, but I couldn't help thinking differently.

On one hand, I knew that if his body changed dramatically then it wouldn't affect how I felt about him, but I also knew men were different. They are much more visual. Even if it didn't change how he saw me, then I was sure it would change how I felt about myself.

I've always had a high sex drive and Steven and I were well matched in that respect. I didn't know how these operations would change things.

It was all very difficult and very real. However, I knew what I had to do. I had to have the surgeries.

Yoga For Releasing Emotional Tension

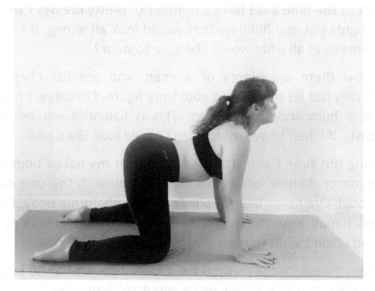

Cat/Cow Stretch

Pose:

Cat/Cow Stretch: On hands and knees with your fingers spread wide and wrists under shoulders, hips over knees. Inhale, lift your heart and hips to the ceiling, exhale, round forward and draw your belly in. Repeat as many times as needed to relieve tension in the neck, shoulders and spine. This can be performed seated, just hold on to your knees to roll through your spine.

Breathing:

Lion's Breath: This can be practiced seated, but I like to do this on my hands and knees. Take a few regular breaths and feel your whole body, notice where the tension is. Now take a deep inhale through your nose, when you exhale open your mouth as wide as you can and stick your tongue out. Make the 'Ha' sound as loud as you can. This is 'Lion's Breath', a great way to relieve tension in the mind and body. Take a few regular breaths in between and 'roar' as many times as you need to.

Meditation:

Healing Light: In child's pose (see Chapter 1), as your head rests on the floor or block, breathe into the centre of your forehead (your third eye). Feel the colour indigo flood into your forehead and clear your mind. When your mind is calm, visualise this healing light through your body to your toes. Stay here for at least 5 minutes.

Chapter 7: The Great Nipple Debate

I felt I was finally getting somewhere after over a year of confusion. I knew I was going to have my ovaries and my breasts removed. For the most part I felt good about potentially saving my life.

I was happy with the department I was under at Hospital O who were going to remove my ovaries. I was just waiting for a date for surgery. I hoped it wouldn't be too long. In one way I wanted it all over and done with, in another way I dreaded them calling.

I was also happy I had found Mr H to perform my breast surgery. I had an appointment to see Mr J, the surgeon who would be removing my breast tissue. I was organised. This made me feel stronger in a strange way.

Steven came with me to my appointment with Mr J on the other side of London. This is a very old and dilapidated hospital, but I was assured my actual surgery would be at Hospital B.

We were led in to the room by a nurse who told me to strip from the waist up and lay on the bed. Mr J would be in to see me soon. The room was boiling hot, smelly and depressing. All hospital rooms are depressing but this was more so than most. As I had already seen Mr H I hoped this appointment was a formality and that we might even talk about dates for surgery.

There I was laying back with my top off and in walked Mr J. He looked like a character from a 'Carry On' film with his bow tie and glasses. He was a highly regarded surgeon and Mr H trusted him and I trusted Mr H.

Very unusually Mr J sat next to me on the bed. Yes, he actually sat on the bed and held my hand. I looked at Steven and he just shrugged his shoulders. Mr J then took my hand in his and then looked into my eyes. He stroked my hand and then told me he was very sorry for my situation.

I felt very exposed and very naked. He examined my breasts and explained that he had worked with Mr H for a long time and they had performed many operations together. He went through my family history (yes again!) and asked me how I felt about losing my breasts.

It was all so strange and so irregular that I burst in to tears. Before or since I have not cried inside a hospital but I couldn't hold it together. I can usually compose myself but I lost control. As I cried Mr J gave me more sympathy which made me cry even more. I'm much better when I'm just faced with the facts.

He explained that the removal of my breasts was a long and lengthy process. I would have a mammogram today and then if all was well I would come back to see him in a few months to discuss things further. I would also need to see a psychologist to see if I was in the right mental state for surgery. Great – I clearly hadn't made a good impression on that front as I had been crying for most of the appointment. He would definitely think I was unstable.

Mr J also informed me of what I now refer to as 'the great nipple debate'. To keep or not to keep – that it the question. Keeping the nipples is not always an option. They literally have to scoop out as much tissue as possible to prevent cancer.

Often this was too much, the nipples died and then had to be removed. Some studies also reported that keeping the nipples slightly increased the risk of getting cancer. That's right – I could go through all this and still get breast cancer as it is impossible to remove all the tissue.

If the nipples are removed they reconstruct false ones by tattooing and making the pointy part of the nipple from another part of your body. Images of plasticine came to mind. The thought of losing my nipples would haunt me.

I was disappointed as I hoped we would be talking about dates, but it now seemed that months of appointments lay ahead and I needed to convince them that I was ready. I wasn't even sure if I was ready, but I knew I needed to push myself forward.

The only encouraging part of the consultation was that Mr J said that it was much easier to recover from the operation when healthy tissue was being removed as opposed to cancerous tissue. As I was fit and healthy then it should mean that I would recover well. This was something my Dad had also said. If I waited for the cancer to come, then recovery (if at all) would obviously be much more difficult.

I was strangely numb when we left that appointment. Sore from the mammogram, I had done all my crying. I just felt lost in the system and helpless. Steven and I had a big row as he said that they probably wouldn't operate for a long time as I cried in the consultation. I wanted to hit him! Of course I was upset – signing up to lose parts of your body makes you feel that way. He didn't mean to upset me, but it played on my mind that I may have postponed things.

Up until that point I had made myself hold it all together in front of my parents, family, friends and work colleagues. I even joked about it some of the time. I was careful that nobody scratched the surface as I didn't know what would happen if they did.

This is my nature. I'm the strong one. But outside that hospital I could feel the mask coming off. I could feel myself sinking.

Yoga To Energise

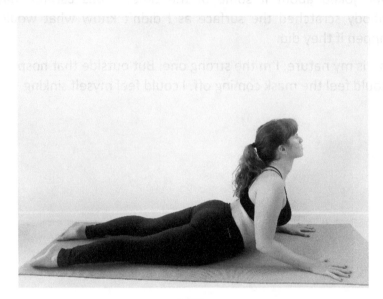

Cobra

Pose:

Cobra: Lay on your tummy with your hands underneath your shoulders. If you have a sore lower back, you can walk your hands further forward. Spread your fingers wide and make sure your legs are hip distance apart. Press your legs into the mat and at the same time press your hands down so that your shoulders lift from the mat. Keep your elbows bent and hug them into your rib cage. Move your shoulders away from your ears and gently draw your shoulder blades together. Hold for 3 breaths and then lower back down. Repeat 5 times. When coming out of the pose, push yourself onto your knees. It may feel good to do Cat/Cow stretch (Chapter 6).

Breathing:

Breath Of Fire: This breathing practice energises your digestive system and tones your tummy. Sit on the floor. Place your hands on the floor and position slightly behind your hips. Sit as tall as you can. Close your eyes. Take a normal breath in and normal breath out then inhale half way. Now take short, sharp exhales through your nose. As you do this pump your belly out. Don't worry about the inhale, this will happen naturally. Try to pump the belly as fast as you can. Build up to 100 breaths over time.

Meditation:

Recharge: It is important to recharge so we don't get depleted. When dealing with a stressful situation I often feel frazzled. Sit or lay comfortably. As you breathe deeply, say silently to yourself 'There is enough time, I have what I need, everything will get done, there is enough time'. Repeat until you feel energised.

Chapter 8: Analyse Me

I knew I wouldn't get a date for breast surgery until I saw the psychologist. Chasing appointments in this situation is difficult. You get transferred from one department to another and put on hold again and again.

Eventually, after 2 months the appointment came through to see the psychologist. My feelings about this were mixed. In one way it would be nice to talk to someone away from family or friends. In another way I didn't want him to class me as psychologically unstable and deny me surgery.

I have a degree in psychology so know quite a lot about therapy and the stages of acceptance. To a certain extent I had been counselling myself for a while, so I thought I was prepped for my appointment. I hoped that this councillor would be different to the genetic counsellors I had seen previously.

Now, I know some people may say that my anger towards some of the professionals I saw at the start of my experience was 'transference'. This is when you can't handle the truth, so your anger and frustration gets vented onto the person who is giving you the bad news. This didn't happen with me. The professionals that I saw at the first hospital were just cold and uncaring.

I turned up at Hospital B for my appointment with the psychologist with an open mind. A tall, lanky man with glasses (yes, the stereotypical look of a psychologist) came to get me from the waiting room. He apologised for being late. It was only by a minute! This is very rare. I've since learnt that you can sit in waiting rooms for hours and hours and you never get an apology. You don't actually care by that point – you're just so pleased to see someone.

Anyway, Mr P seemed friendly enough and he made me feel at ease instantly. As I explained what had happened to me up to this point Mr P was very shocked that I hadn't been offered counselling about the imminent removal of my ovaries. He said we could talk about this too if I wanted.

We obviously spoke about my family history (as you know that's a given in any appointment), but he quickly moved forward to how I felt about it all. I was honest that I was scared and that trying to manage family and friends' feelings as well can be very draining. Mr P told me something I already knew but I'm not very good at following – 'You don't have to be strong all the time'.

Hearing a stranger say this made an impact. Maybe it was okay to admit that this situation was crap and at times I found it hard to cope with the way my life was changing.

I told Mr P about wanting to get all my surgeries over by the end of 2016. It was March 2016 at this point and he said that seemed reasonable to him. I was still waiting for my ovary surgery date so things were still up in the air.

He asked me to fill out a form which at first glance I thought was a bit of a waste of time, but by the end of the session I saw the value. I basically had to rate on a scale of one to ten how important the key issues we spoke about were:

- Nipple conservation (10)
- Operation by the end of 2016 (10)
- To be in hospital for the shortest amount of time (10)

- Keep breasts the same size (8)
- Maintaining flexibility for teaching yoga (10)
- Maintaining sex life, also in relation to HRT (10)
- To be able to wear tight fitting clothes (8)
- To be able to wear a bikini (8)

He told me that my case would be presented in front of professionals and reviewed. Mr P said that in his opinion I was psychologically ready for surgery. I didn't know if he was right, but I hoped he was!

Mr P told me about a support group which meets at the hospital every few months for women in my situation. Some women will even show you the results of their surgeries. I'm sure this helps many ladies but for me the thought of sitting round talking about the gene mutation and surgeries was not for me. I also couldn't bear to see the results of surgery. I simply didn't want to have any expectations.

Of course there were horror pictures in my mind. I thought that if I saw good results of surgery then this would raise my hopes and if I saw bad results then this would scare me even more. I resisted the urge to look at pictures online and instead hoped for the best.

Mr P told me that I could come back and see him at any time, but that he wasn't going to make it compulsory. Did this mean I was psychologically stable or had I just held it together in the session? I wasn't sure, but I did feel like I was getting somewhere in the process.

Having this gene mutation is such a tangle of emotions. You need to deal with thinking about your mortality; you question if you are still going to feel like a woman without your breasts and ovaries; mourn your loss of fertility and accept going through the menopause. Each one of these has a huge psychological impact and when you put them together it is very hard to cope.

The constant that helped me keep my head together was my daily yoga practice. I know this sounds sugar coated but it's true. So I kept doing the thing that cleared my head like no other and I just carried on.

Yoga For Clear Thinking

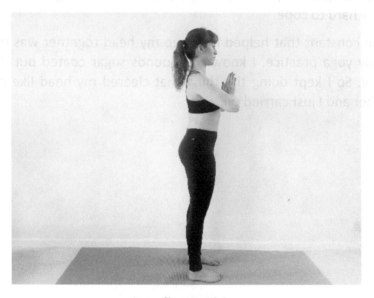

Standing Position

Pose:

<u>Half Sun Salutations</u>: This short sequence stimulates the body and awakens the mind.

- Standing position: Stand tall with your feet hip distance apart and parallel, knees slightly bent, belly drawn in, shoulders rolled back and hands together in front of your heart.
- Inhale to lift your arms overhead. Try to keep your rib cage drawn into your body.

- Exhale to fold forward. Hinge from your hips and keep your back flat as you fold. Bend your knees as much as you need to. End in a forward fold (Chapter 3).
- Inhale and place your hands on your shins and lengthen your spine. Look ahead. This is Half Way Lift.
- Exhale to a forward fold.
- Inhale roll through your spine to come up to a standing position with your arms overhead.
- Exhale bring your hands together in front of your heart.

Repeat 5 times.

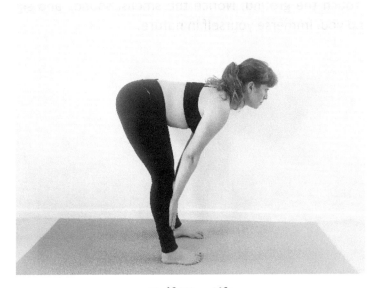

Half Way Lift

Breathing:

Mind Cleanse: This really clears my mind. Inhale with a full breath for the count of 4, hold the breath for 4, exhale for the count of 4, hold your lungs empty for the count of 4. Repeat until you feel calm.

Meditation:

Walking Meditation: Sometimes I find the best way to clear my mind is to get outside in the fresh air. Try to turn off your phone for 10 minutes so you can concentrate. If it is appropriate walk barefoot. Notice how your feet feel when they touch the ground. Notice the smells, sounds and sights around you. Immerse yourself in nature.

Chapter 9: Getting The Date

In March 2016 I finally got the call for the date of my ovary and fallopian tube surgery. I was in the car on the way back from work with Steven. This was the call I had been hoping for but as the lady told me the date of surgery, 6th July 2016, I completely froze. I managed to take down the details and she asked me if I was prepared to be put on the waiting list for a cancellation which I agreed. The sooner this was all over the better as far as I was concerned.

Now I knew the date I could get my life in order. I could organise things at work and more importantly I could tell my breast surgeons and hopefully move forward to schedule that operation.

I felt quite numb after getting the date. Some inner strength was helping me to keep pushing ahead with my decision and on the surface I was as strong as ever. However, inside I was suffering.

As you know I had collapsed months earlier, and although this hadn't happened again, I was still experiencing dizzy spells. I was also finding it hard to sleep as when I did I had horrific nightmares. These nightmares included me losing parts of my body and also being lost in different scenarios. They were very real and very scary.

In retrospect, I was also completely exhausted. I was teaching a lot of yoga classes and my job at Studio 666 was demanding. My boss would disappear for months at a time on one personal crisis or another then turn up and pick holes in whatever had happened in her absence. This was frustrating as I kept the studio running smoothly and I generated a lot of income, but nothing was ever good enough. Although she knew about my situation she never once asked me about my health, she just moaned about the tiny problems in her own life.

My colleagues on the other hand thought nothing of asking me 'if I was keeping my nipples or not' and probed me for information as often as they could. This was a really hostile environment with lots of back stabbing, so their constant questions made it even worse. I was working in the office 3 days a week and although I tried to keep my head down and carry on it was impossible. Thankfully my boss agreed to me working from home 2 days a week, so this took the pressure off slightly.

I knew that if I didn't do something to stop my nightmares I might collapse again. My friend suggested a therapist she had used who had stopped her nightmares. She gives treatments of Craniosacral Therapy. I had never heard of it before, but I was willing to try anything at that point.

My first session was incredible. G is a softly spoken lady with eyes that see right through you. My friend had joked and referred to her as a 'white witch' and I could see why. She just has an air of magic about her and I felt immediately at ease.

I sat down and told her everything. By then it had been a year and a half since I had found out I had the gene mutation. I completely poured my heart out with everything from problems in my relationship, to struggling with the travel to Leeds each week, to my upcoming operations, to my work – it all came flooding out. She listened patiently. I realised I had in fact been through a lot already and I should give myself a break. I wasn't superwoman. It was okay if I felt exhausted and upset.

When I had finished talking she asked me to lay on the bed. G then placed her hands on different parts of my body from my feet to my head. To this day I do not understand Craniosacral Therapy. Of course, I could Google it but I prefer not to. I like to think it is magic. Magic that feels amazing!

That night I slept well for the first time in ages. I awoke feeling less frazzled and far more rested. I still see G for treatments and she has helped me greatly. Now I know I'm a bit alternative and this type of treatment might not be for everyone but it worked for me.

I could have gone back to see the psychologist, but I never did. He was great but this alternative therapy felt right. At least I could sleep better and I was more relaxed. I wasn't in the office with the bitches any more. I realised I had to give myself a bit more 'me' time. I made time to have baths and to go swimming which I love. I also started reading novels again – another thing I enjoy that slipped away due to lack of time.

I was in a better place - I now just had to mentally prepare myself for surgery.

Yoga For Anxiety

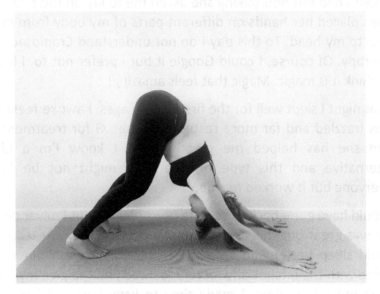

Downward Facing Dog

Pose:

<u>Downward Facing Dog</u>: This is a great anxiety reliever, providing you ample time to rest your mind and stretch out tense muscles. Begin in a standing position (Chapter 8) and exhale as you bend into a forward fold (Chapter 3). Bend your knees more so you can place your palms on the mat, shoulder width apart, with your fingers spread wide. Step your legs back, so you make an inverted V shape with your body, feet hip distance apart. Keep a soft bend in your knees and gently press your chest towards your thighs. Breathe slowly for 60 seconds and repeat for ultimate relief. It can be good to practice cat/cow (Chapter 6) after downward facing dog.

Breathing:

Bumblebee Breath: Close your throat slightly so you can hear your breath when you breathe in. Cover your ears with your thumbs and your eyes with your fingers. Keep your lips closed lightly and your teeth slightly apart with your jaw relaxed. Breathe out slowly making a low humming sound. Make your exhalation long and smooth. Repeat for 2 minutes.

Meditation:

Picture Perfect: Find a picture you love and which calms you. It can be a lovely painting, a clipping from a magazine or holiday brochure. It can be a photo of you, your family or friends having a great time. Any picture that makes you feel good. Breathe deeply whilst looking at it. Study the images, colours and shadows. Feel your mind calming down. Look at this picture whenever you feel anxious.

Chapter 10: Preparation

To make things even more chaotic my Dad needed an operation on his back and this was scheduled a couple of days before my surgery. Everything always happens together!

Two days before my own operation, I spent the day in the hospital with my Dad. As he was being operated on privately I expected there to be no delays and great service. Instead he was kept waiting all day and by the time he had surgery was very hungry and severely dehydrated.

I was more nervous about my Dad's operation than any of my own. He had dreadful sciatica and he could barely walk without terrible pain. I was so scared that something would go wrong in the operation and he wouldn't be able to walk.

Fortunately, the operation went well but the aftercare in the private hospital was appalling. The nurses were nowhere to be seen and we were scared to leave him overnight as nobody seemed to care.

The day before my surgery we went to visit my Dad in hospital. He looked well and was already walking around which was a huge relief.

However, the strain of that long day caused an argument between me and Steven. I can't remember the details but he said he was going home. At that point I thought it may be for the best. I could then just focus on getting through the operation and not have to worry about arguing with him.

He was set to leave but then I received a phone call. It was from the hospital informing me that my operation had been postponed due to my low resting heart rate. Apparently, they wanted to run more tests.

I completely lost control and cried like a baby. All the work I had done preparing myself and getting in 'the right place' would be for nothing. Plus there was absolutely nothing wrong with me. As I am fit, my resting heart rate is naturally low. If they had bothered to read my notes they would have realised this.

My Mum and Steven tried to console me but they couldn't. I was broken. I managed to speak to a supervisor and begged her to ask the head anaesthetist to look through my notes again. We all sat there anxiously waiting for the phone to ring.

Fortunately, when they called back they agreed that I was fit for surgery and I could come in tomorrow as planned. I felt a mixture of relief and nerves. I wanted to get it over with but the whole thing just felt so final. No chance of children ever.

I knew I didn't want children but on the early morning tube ride to the hospital the following day I kept asking myself if I was sure. As a former primary school teacher I had been fond of many children – maybe I did want them or at least the chance to change my mind in the future. Even up to the last minutes before surgery I was asking myself these questions. I didn't share these thoughts with Steven as most of them didn't make sense even in my head.

Many people have asked me if I get nervous before an operation. The best way I can describe it is like being at the top of a cliff, knowing you must jump and needing to find the courage to do it.

I took a deep breath and jumped.

| Yoga To Prepare For Surgery |

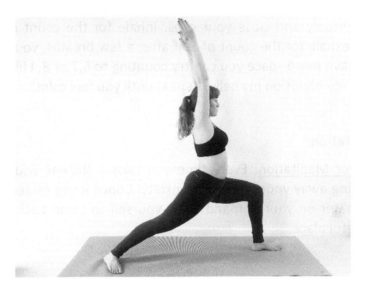

Warrior 1

Pose:

Warrior 1: Warrior poses induce strength and focus in the body and mind. Begin in a strong standing position (Chapter 8) with your feet hip distance. Take a long step back with your right foot and place your heel on the floor. Your left toes will point forward and your right toes will turn out to a 45 degree angle. With your hands on your hips, gently swing your right hip forward so the hips are square. Keep your right leg straight and strong and bend your left knee. Make sure your knee does not go over your ankle, if it does take a small step forward. If you feel stable reach your arms overhead with the palms facing and soften your shoulders. Hold for 5 breaths then step your right foot forward to the top of the mat. Repeat stepping your left foot back.

Breathing:

Peaceful Breath: This is very simple, but I found it highly effective for calming nerves before surgery. Sit or lay comfortably and close your eyes. Inhale for the count of 5, then exhale for the count of 5. If after a few breaths, you feel you have more space you can try counting to 6,7 or 8. I like to place my hands on my belly. Repeat until you feel calm.

Meditation:

Shower Meditation: Every time you take a shower visualise washing away your stress and anxiety. Concentrate on feeling the water on your skin and allow yourself to come back to a peaceful place.

Chapter 11: Recovery

I came round to the sound of bleeping machines and the acrid hospital smell. The nurse told me that everything had gone well. I tentatively touched my tummy and realised that it was very bloated. It might have been my imagination, but it felt very empty too.

As the nurse left to attend to another patient I placed both hands on my belly, closed my eyes and began to breathe deeply. I knew that I needed to get as much breath into this area as possible to help me recover. After a few minutes I felt calmer and more aware.

My main aim was to get home as quickly as possible – I didn't want to stay the night. I was desperate for the toilet but I wouldn't use the bed pan. Instead I convinced the nurse to escort me to the toilet. I felt nauseous and unsteady but I told the nurse I was okay. She left me in the toilet cubicle unaided so I carefully pulled up my hospital gown so I could see my tummy. It was red, swollen and the bruising was starting to show. The incisions were small and neat, one just under my belly button and two further ones near my hip bones. I took a few more deep breaths.

When I came out of the toilet the nurse had gone. I forced myself to walk around a little as I knew this would help me to get over the anaesthetic quicker. Eventually I got ushered back to bed and I asked to see Steven. They said I couldn't as I was still in the recovery room, but as soon as a bed became available then I could see him on the ward. I sat there having the obligatory tea and biscuits (I actually brought my own peppermint tea – God the nurses must have hated me!) and I waited.

An hour went by and there was still no news of a bed. Eventually they let Steven in. By this point I was sitting up and feeling much stronger. The relief on his face was huge and now I had my phone I could talk to my parents.

As Steven sat on the bed and cuddled me, I remembered the moments before I went through to theatre which were really hard for both of us. Steven walked me down with the porter as far as he was allowed and gave me a big hug. As I walked away from him my legs were shaking and I wanted to cry, but I had to hold it together. I thought that if they saw me upset they might not operate on me at all.

We also talked about the great relief of life with no more period pains. I had suffered the monthly indescribable cramps for as long as I could remember. I really couldn't imagine how amazing it would be without them.

Added to this, for the last year I also had a contraceptive copper coil. This had given me dreadful pain. After a few accidents with condoms I decided this was the best way not to get pregnant. Having a coil fitted is the most horrific experience. Apparently, it's not as bad if you have had children but obviously this wasn't the case for me. I went through this pain twice as the first time the doctor inserted the coil in the wrong place.

Over the previous months the coil had become very painful – just like a tampon that's moved around and become uncomfortable. During the surgery they removed it and I asked to keep it. I wanted to see the thing that had given me such grief. I sat there with the coil in a plastic container and rattled it around. I couldn't believe it was so tiny.

After a few hours stuck in the recovery room, they needed the space and I needed to go home. I quickly dressed and armed with my bag of painkillers left the hospital. I was so hungry and I really wanted a burger. I eat healthily most of the time and very rarely have this type of food but that's what I fancied. Sitting outside in the hot summer sunshine greedily eating my burger, fries and strawberry milkshake I felt good. I felt relieved. One step was over. I still had to wait for the standard biopsy of the tissue that had been removed but at least the operation was finished.

The thought of sitting in a cab for over an hour to travel across London was not appealing so we got on the tube. Steven and my parents didn't think this was a good idea but I insisted. Steven stood in front of me so I wouldn't get pushed. It was just good to be out of the hospital and not staying in overnight.

By the time I got home the painkillers had started to wear off and the bruising was more vivid. Ironically, I looked pregnant as I was so bloated.

It was good to get home and my Dad was set to arrive home from hospital the following day, so everything was working out. I felt strangely energised but got tired very quickly. After a nap, Steven and I did what I made him promise me before surgery, we had sex. Now I know that sounds crazy to have sex the same day as surgery but it was really important to me.

The removal of my ovaries didn't just signal the end of my fertility, but it also could mean the loss of my sex drive which has always been healthy. More than anything else I just wanted to feel 'normal'. I didn't want to feel dried up and old at the age of 38.

Steven really didn't think it was a good idea but I insisted we try. It hurt a lot as all my internal muscles had tensed up during the surgery, but I wanted to keep trying. I had this idea in my head that if I didn't have sex then I never would again. It was extremely uncomfortable but at least I felt normal.

I slept deeply, knocked out by painkillers and awoke feeling sore and bloated but okay. I wanted to carry on with my yoga practice so I rolled out my mat. I didn't really know what I should be doing but I just knew I had to move and breathe.

My practice focussed on simple breathing exercises, gentle leg stretches and hip openers. I avoided twists, backbends and laying on my front. I felt better after my 20 minutes on the mat.

That day I was scheduled to see Mr J about my breast surgery. I tried to change the date but the next available appointment was in four months' time. I was told by Mr J that I had to keep the appointment so that my name was near the top of the list. I didn't want them to forget about me.

I took strong painkillers and took the tube with Steven to the other side of London. I just hoped someone didn't knock into me and bang my sore tummy. It was a boiling hot day and it took an hour and a half to get to the hospital.

I felt disorientated. I rarely take painkillers so I felt dizzy and sick. My tummy was very painful.

The whole episode was a complete waste of time. I waited ages to see Mr J. He didn't even acknowledge that I must be in a considerable amount of pain as I'd had surgery the day before. He labelled the removal of my ovaries and fallopian tubes as 'the easy part' of the process.

It's true the ovary surgery is more straightforward, but it definitely didn't feel 'easy' to me. He examined me again and told me that I was still on the waiting list. He said my operation may be in the autumn or even next year.

I really wanted to keep to my self-imposed schedule of getting both ops over in the same year. To me it made sense – just have one crap year then move on. However, I was in their hands so I just had to hope for the best.

On the way home we broke the journey up by having lunch in Leicester Square. At this point, I had decided that I wasn't going to take any more painkillers. I could cope better with the discomfort than the queasy feeling from the drugs.

The next few days were a bit of a blur of pain and trying to get on with things as normally as possible. My Dad was making a great recovery too and this was a weight off my mind. Steven and I busied ourselves buying furniture for my new apartment which I was set to move into in the coming weeks. Everything felt like it was shifting and changing. I carried on practicing gentle yoga daily. It really helped me feel more grounded. After my burger blip, I also tried to eat well to aid my recovery.

I had booked a canal boat trip for Steven's birthday before I got the date for my surgery. So just four days after surgery we travelled to Sowerby Bridge, Yorkshire for the trip. I thought about cancelling but it was non-refundable and the break would probably do me good.

Neither of us had been on a canal boat before and we had great fun trying to steer and navigate the locks. Steven took care of the heavy work as I wouldn't be able to lift anything for a few months yet. It was great being in the beautiful countryside and I found this really healing. I even wore a bikini, not worrying about showing my unsightly belly. As well as gentle daily yoga I started to do other exercise. I was careful but realised quickly I could gently jog and build strength in my arms and legs. I just had to avoid core work.

Sex was still uncomfortable and to make matters worse I had this horrible smelly discharge. I had never felt so unattractive. I had a huge bloated, bruised tummy and I felt fat. Steven did his best to reassure me that he still found me attractive, but it's all about how you feel inside.

I knew my body would heal, but I also knew that this would be the easy part. My mind and soul had to heal too.

Yoga To Aid Recovery

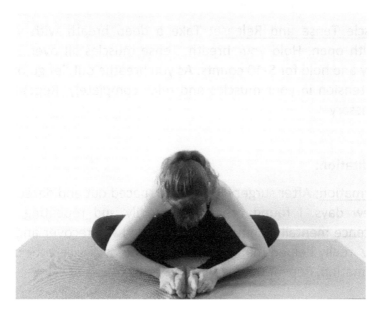

Seated Butterfly

Pose:

Seated Butterfly: Sit on a cushion or block and bring the soles of your feet together and let your knees drop open. Place your hands on the floor behind your hips and sit tall. This may be enough of a stretch or you can creep your hands forward in front of you. Gently draw your shoulder blades together and encourage your shoulders away from your ears. Now you can relax your head downwards. Breathe deeply. Stay until you feel your hips and lower back release.

Breathing:

I found I had a lot of tension throughout my whole body after surgery and this exercise really helped.

<u>Muscle Tense and Release</u>: Take a deep breath with your mouth open. Hold your breath. Tense muscles all over your body and hold for 5-10 counts. As you breathe out, let go of all the tension in your muscles and relax completely. Repeat as necessary.

Meditation:

<u>Affirmation</u>: After surgery I felt quite spaced out and dazed for a few days. I found breathing steadily and repeating the sentence mentally 'I am calm, I am safe, I will recover and be okay' really helped me. You can use mine or create your own affirmation. Repeat until you feel clear headed and calm.

Chapter 12: One Down, One To Go

By the following month, the bloating in my belly had gone down enough for me to fit back into my jeans. The bruising on my tummy was also disappearing and the scars less angry.

At my check up, the consultant couldn't believe how well I had healed. I think this was due to daily yoga, gentle exercise and eating well. It's not rocket science but often when you are in the middle of a stressful time it's easy to forget. I was lucky that before this whole drama started I had a healthy lifestyle which made me feel good. I simply carried on and that led me to recovery. The hospital also gave me the fantastic news that the biopsy result was normal, meaning there was no cancer detected.

It was very strange not having a monthly cycle ticking away in the background. I always knew when I was ovulating and when I was about to get my period. I cried as I threw away my remaining tampons, but at the same time it was hugely liberating.

Steven and I took a short trip to Scarborough. The weather was great and we saw Bryan Adams in concert. I was more relaxed than I had been for ages.

On the morning we were due to leave, I got a phone call from Hospital B with a date for my breast surgery. I was to lose my breasts on 26th October 2016. I was a jumble of emotions.

Steven quickly checked his diary and realised he had gigs the week of my surgery. As a musician, work is hard to come by, but I felt upset that I wasn't his number one priority. I know he didn't mean to be this way, but men can be very selfish at times. I told him that he didn't need to be there for my surgery, but he insisted.

I felt good that everything was organised and I had a date in place. One of the hardest things I found about this process is the constant feeling of being in limbo, waiting for surgery dates.

For the next few months my work at Studio 666 dominated. It was very frustrating as it seemed the harder I worked the less my boss appreciated me. The times when I did have to go into the office for meetings I was probed about my situation. I knew they thought I was strange for not wanting children.

In fact, this has been a constant throughout my adult life. I've had friends who have talked about nothing else apart from 'settling down' and 'breeding'. I could never identify with this as there was always so many other things that seemed more interesting. Also thinking about that way of life made me feel trapped and uncomfortable.

However, although I have always supported their choice, I have often been branded 'strange', 'unfeminine', 'going against nature' or 'there must be something wrong with you'. To make matters worse, when friends married and started a family they didn't want to know me anymore as I didn't fit the mould. They wanted to hang out with friends who had children, so the friendship soon drifted apart.

The spiteful ladies at Studio 666 were no exception They made me feel unnatural and that there was something wrong with me. They made a difficult time of my life so much worse and I wanted more than anything to leave.

Unfortunately, it wasn't that easy due to my lifestyle with Steven. By this point he was sharing the travel with me, but in reality, I only had between Wednesday to Saturday in London to earn a living. My work at Studio 666 fitted in perfectly. I could work remotely some of the time and then when in London I could teach yoga classes.

I still really enjoyed teaching but most of the time I was so burnt out from my work at Studio 666, I didn't give my best in classes. I had visions of setting up a small yoga studio of my own, but I couldn't see how that would work as I wasn't in one place all the time. I also didn't have the funds and felt that I couldn't start anything new until these operations were behind me. I was dependent on waiting for dates. I felt like I couldn't move on and felt incredibly claustrophobic.

I had no choice but to keep my head down and get on with things. I just hoped that after my operation I could make a change.

During the next few months my belly became less bloated and the bruising disappeared. I was left with a slight paunch. I didn't like it as I'd always had a flat tummy. After doing some reading online I found out that it takes about two years for your tummy to go back to normal after the removal of ovaries. I didn't want to wait this long, so when I felt I had healed internally I started daily abdominal exercises to speed up the process. I also practiced the breathing exercise 'Breath of Fire' (Chapter 7).

Initially my consultant had told me that because of my age I would need to be on HRT for at least 10 years. This was to protect my bones and heart. I don't like taking tablets, but in my situation, I knew I didn't have a choice. So after the operation I started the medication.

For the first month or so I experienced some hot flushes. It felt like someone pouring boiling water inside me but only lasted for a few minutes. I also had the occasional night sweat. Both of these were manageable and definitely not as bad as I had expected. I still had the same sex drive and hadn't dried up like a prune.

All in all, I was thrilled with the result. I had thought that the moment I woke up after surgery I would have automatically aged 10 years but I didn't, I still felt like me.

Sex wasn't painful anymore and after a few weeks the discharge went. I wish somebody had told me about this side of things. I had no idea what to expect and no idea what was 'normal'.

I felt stronger and healthier. I just had to now prepare myself for breast surgery. Fortunately, I had more exciting things to think about. It was a 'big birthday' for my Dad so Steven and I were going on holiday with my parents. It was a trip of a lifetime. We flew to Toronto, travelled to Niagara Falls and then New York. From here we boarded the Queen Mary 2 and sailed all the way back to Southampton.

The trip came at exactly the right time and it's what we all needed. We saw amazing places and had fantastic food. Every now and then I thought about the upcoming breast surgery, but for the most part it didn't cross my mind. I arrived home happy, healthy and relaxed.

Yoga For Increasing Determination

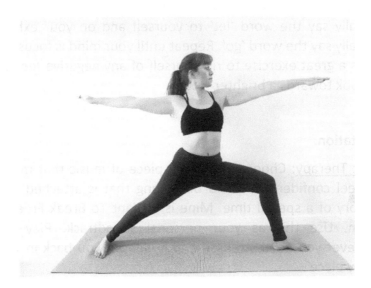

Warrior 2

Pose:

Warrior 2: This pose brings determination and focus into mind and body. Stand with your feet slightly wider than your hips and your hands on your hips. Remember the standing principles in Chapter 8. Turn your right foot out 90 degrees and angle your left foot in 20 degrees. Make sure your right heel is aligned with the arch of your left foot. Gently lift your right hip up so it is in line with your left hip. Keep your left leg straight and strong then bend your right knee. If your knee comes past your ankle then make your stance wider. If you feel stable, reach your arms to shoulder height and look towards your right fingertips. Hold for 5 breaths then straighten your right leg and turn your toes back to centre. Repeat on the left side.

Breathing:

Let Go: Find a comfortable position. Close your eyes and begin to breathe deeply through your nose. On each inhale, mentally say the word 'let' to yourself and on your exhale, mentally say the word 'go'. Repeat until your mind is focussed. This is a great exercise to rid yourself of any negative feelings and look towards a brighter future.

Meditation:

Music Therapy: Choose an upbeat piece of music that makes you feel confident. It could be a song that is attached to a memory of a special time. Mine is 'I Want To Break Free' by Queen. Use this as your personal soundtrack. Play this whenever you need strength and it will put you back in your 'happy place'.

Chapter 13: Staying Calm

Finally, the day of my breast surgery came. I had physically and mentally prepared myself. I had eaten well, exercised and had sessions with my healer. My apartment was clean and my bag was packed. I had organised cover for my classes and my work at Studio 666 was up to date. It felt like I was going on holiday, I'd even had my eyelashes tinted. I felt calm, I felt well.

The night before surgery I feel like I need to go into a little hole. I don't want to speak to anyone other than Steven and my parents. I make sure all the 'well-wisher' calls happen in the previous days. I need some quiet time so I do some gentle yoga then watch a cheesy chick flick. I also burn white sage which helps with any new journey ahead and if possible try to get a good night's sleep.

The surgery would take several hours and with any operation there are risks. There was always a chance that I wouldn't come round from the surgery. I made Steven promise to look out for my parents if I didn't make it.

It was a cold, foggy morning as my Dad dropped Steven and me to Brixton tube station. It was decided that my parents would travel up later as only one person could come with me into the surgical admission area. Holding hands, we walked past the Electric Avenue neon sign that always makes me smile as the song runs through my head. I love London.

As we walked up the hill towards Hospital B, I made sure I took big deep breaths. I knew that I would be stuck with the stale hospital atmosphere for the next few days. The fog was thicker here with the smell of autumn in the air and feel of Halloween around made me feel cosy.

We registered and sat waiting in the hot waiting room/corridor at 7:30am. My last drink of water was 5am so I was already thirsty from the journey. I looked on as Steven swigged from a bottle of water. Hopefully I wouldn't be waiting long, I just wanted it over.

We only waited for a few minutes before I was called by a nurse to do my obs and attach my hospital bracelets – one on each wrist. As I changed into my hospital gown and surgical stockings, I looked at my breasts for the last time. I didn't know how I was going to look afterwards. The previous night before my shower I had mentally said goodbye to this part of my body. I just had to be brave and jump off the cliff again.

Sitting in the corridor, the hospital gown rubbed against my nipples. I wondered if I would ever feel this sensation again or if I would have nipples at all. In a previous appointment I had with one of Mr H's registrars he told me that if my nipples could be spared then there would probably be no feeling at all. My nipples have always been very sensitive which is a sensation I enjoyed. It was hard to imagine never feeling this again.

Quickly I was ushered into a room with one of Mr H's registrars. He completed my paperwork and then Mr H and two other registrars joined us. Mr H examined me and drew some lines on my chest. He is such a great man. He instantly puts you at ease and always makes eye contact. Even though he is very busy he gives you as much time as you need. I explained again how important it was for me to save my nipples and he explained that he would do everything possible. He told me I was first on the list so I would be in theatre shortly. It was all going to plan.

We sat back in the waiting corridor, my heart beating wildly. I was strangely buzzing with all the adrenaline coursing through my body. It wouldn't be long now, it was going to happen. I called my parents to let them know.

We waited and waited and then waited some more. I knew that there must be something wrong. I didn't know what to think. Eventually a harassed Mr H came to find us and led us into a small stuffy room. His team of registrars followed. He told us that Mr J had not turned up for my surgery and they couldn't locate him. Without Mr J the surgery couldn't go ahead. He was removing the breast tissue and Mr H was reconstructing. The room began to spin, I felt sick.

Mr H gave me two options – we could either reschedule or use another surgeon who was in the hospital that day for a meeting. He had agreed in principle to operate on me. I had never met him. I was so ready for this to be done. I asked Mr H if he trusted this new surgeon, Mr G, and he said that he was excellent. That was good enough for me so I agreed.

Mr G wanted to meet with me before the surgery as he had some questions. We waited for another hour and a half. By then I didn't know how I was feeling – scared that the operation would still be cancelled – scared that it was still going ahead – I went from one emotion to the other. Eventually Mr G called my name and we went through to another small, stuffy room. He told me that he had read my notes and was willing to operate on me today. I thanked him and liked him instantly. He seemed genuinely concerned.

Apparently somewhere in my notes it was written that I wanted my nipples removed! I told him that I definitely wanted them saved if possible. It didn't inspire me with a great deal of confidence. He also told me that the letter to say that I had the BRCA 1 gene mutation was missing from my file. They were trying to locate it but without that he wouldn't operate on me today.

Dr G had been caught out in the past. He had operated on a lady without seeing the paperwork and it turned out that she didn't have the gene at all. Who would go through all of this if they didn't have the gene mutation?

I remembered that I had a copy of the missing letter at home. My Dad quickly located the letter and emailed it to me. The surgery was back on.

By this time it was about one o'clock. We had been at the hospital since 7am and my last drink of water was 6 hours ago. My last meal was the previous night. I was thirsty, hungry, tired and I'd been through every emotion under the sun. I was completely drained – not the best way to be before a long surgery. As Steven cuddled me, I felt my nipples against his chest. I didn't know if I'd ever feel this again.

I kept busy by walking up and down the corridor, I tried my best to steady my breath. I wanted to keep standing as I would be laying down for a long time. I thought that if I moved around it would help my circulation. We were almost the last people left in the waiting corridor. I was sure the surgery would be cancelled.

Then my name was called. It was half past two. Even though I had been expecting/wanting this for hours it was still a shock. The nurse double checked my name bracelets before handing me a pillow. It seemed that patients now had to carry their own pillow down to surgery. As I hugged Steven, I fought to hold it together. I was exhausted.

I followed the nurse down to theatre and she made the usual upbeat chit chat for which I was grateful. I couldn't help seeing the funny side of my outfit – 2 white surgical gowns, bright red surgical stockings and a white pillow tucked under my arm. It looked like I was going to a fancy dress sleepover!

When I got to the pre-op room, there was loud rock music blaring out. I had met the anaesthetist earlier. She was a pleasant lady with a huge man's Rolex watch on her wrist. As she and two nurses made sure I was comfortable, they carried on the upbeat chatter with me. I'm convinced they all do this to stop you from running. It worked for me. They put stickers on my chest and back, inserted a cannula and removed my gown. I was ready.

My heart felt like it was beating out of my chest, but when I looked at the monitor my pulse was 65 and my blood pressure was 140/75. This was great considering my circumstances.

You should try to look for the good in all situations. I've discovered that my favourite part of operations is the pre-med they give you just before the anaesthetic. The idea is that it relaxes you and I'm sure it has other medical benefits too. It feels amazing. You don't care about a thing. So as the anaesthetic was injected into me I closed my eyes and drifted into a peaceful sleep.

Yoga For Calming The Mind

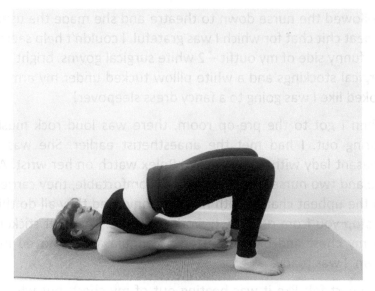

Bridge Pose

Pose:

<u>Bridge Pose</u>: Lay on your back with your knees bent, feet on the floor. Make sure your ankles are underneath your knees and your feet are hip distance apart and parallel. Let your arms relax by your sides. Inhale, press your feet down and lift your bottom away from the floor. Move your shoulder blades closer together and interlock your fingers behind your back, pressing the outer wrists into your mat. Hold here for five breaths activating your legs. Exhale, release your hands and roll down to the floor. Your upper back touches the floor first, then middle back and finally lower back. Repeat 5 times.

Breathing:

<u>4-7-8 Breathing</u>: Place the tip of your tongue against the gums behind your top front teeth. Quietly breathe in through the nose for the count of 4. Hold your breath for the count of 7. Exhale through the mouth making the whooshing sound for the count of 8. Repeat 4 times.

Meditation:

<u>Calming Scents</u>: I use essential oils to change my mood. I like sweet orange and peppermint to energise me, eucalyptus if I'm run down and lavender or camomile to calm me. I also love to burn white sage. The smell instantly soothes me and puts me in a relaxed place. I always take some oils into hospital with me. Find a smell which puts you in a tranquil state of mind. Carry the scent with you and sniff whenever you need to relax.

Chapter 14: Waking Up

What was that pain at the back of my head? As I woke up that's all I could think about. It felt like I had been hit over the head with a blunt object. As I came round, I asked the nurse what had happened to my head. She looked confused and told me that the operation had gone as planned.

I looked down at my chest and realised I had large white tape holding my new breasts in place. At least I had breasts. My chest felt like I had been hit by a ten ton truck but my head was far worse. It was like they had chosen not to anesthetise me but had hit me over the head instead.

As I began to panic and feel sick I urged myself to breathe deeply. I gave myself a few minutes to calm down. I needed to pee desperately so I asked to nurse to help me to the toilet. She said I needed to stay put and use a bed pan. I said that I felt embarrassed. If she just gave me a bit of help to the toilet then I would be okay. She wouldn't listen. I had the choice of either wetting myself as I'd had so many fluids pumped in to me, or using the bed pan, so I choose the latter.

As I raised my hips so she could insert the bed pan under me, shooting pains danced around in my head. Even though I was busting to pee I couldn't. Nobody is used to lying down and peeing apart from the old and infirm. I felt like both at that moment. I hated this loss of dignity.

When the registrar came to see me in the recovery room he also couldn't answer the question about my sore head. He told me that the operation had gone as planned but they had a few problems with my left side as the skin was so thin. I had both my nipples but they could die in the next few weeks and would have to be removed. This often happens as the circulation is poor so the blood can't get to them. I hoped that they would be okay as I didn't want to end up with one nipple. If that was going to be the case I would have them both removed.

I waited a long time in the recovery room as there was no porter to wheel me to the ward. In the end two nurses took me back as it was the end of their shift. Coming out of the lift and rounding the corner, I saw my parents and Steven waiting for me. They asked me how I felt and I told them, 'I've had better days'.

By now it was 10:30pm and the visiting time was over. Luckily the ward sister said that my parents and Steven could stay for a short while. They had been waiting for me to come up to the ward for hours. The ward was hot, dark and depressing. I was told to rest, but I needed to get out of bed. I had been lying down for hours. I realised I wasn't wearing any knickers and felt instantly uncomfortable. Back to the loss of dignity. I quickly instructed my visitors to unpack my bag so I had everything to hand. I felt sick and dizzy but I knew I had to get up.

I had a drip attached to my left hand and a drain coming out from the side of each breast. I tentatively swung my legs over to the side of the bed and began to sit up, taking care not to disturb my drains. Steven helped me to stand and I felt unsteady but forced myself to walk the 10 steps to the toilet. My lower back ached as I had been lying down for so long. I asked Steven to wait outside. I needed to do this myself.

I washed my face, brushed my teeth, brushed my hair, went to the toilet and put my knickers on. Already I felt a little better. I had to know what I looked like so I carefully opened my hospital gown. The thick white tape was stuck across the top part of my breasts, above my nipples. Underneath my breasts, Steri Strips covered the stitches. The bruising was black and blue and even spread towards my belly button. The thing that struck me the most were my nipples. They were black and shrivelled. I couldn't see how they would possibly survive.

As I made my way back to the bed with Steven's help, my heart sank as I realised I would probably lose my nipples. I forced myself to think in a positive way. At least I'd come round from the surgery. Back in bed, my Dad examined the back of my head and found I had a huge bump. I was told that I had to lie on my back for the next 6-8 weeks, but as my head was so painful this was very uncomfortable.

My parents and Steven stayed for as long as they could, but eventually they were ushered out. It had been a very long day for them too and they looked exhausted. As I walked them to the door, with my drip stand in one hand and my drains in a plastic bag in the other, panic set in. I wanted to go home, I didn't want to stay here.

I manged to stay strong during the goodbyes. I clung to Steven a little longer. Then they disappeared into the lift telling me they would be back in the morning. I was all alone.

Yoga For Panic

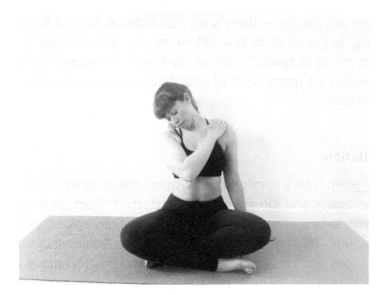

Neck Release

Pose:

<u>Neck Release</u>: This can be performed seated or standing. Place your right hand on your left shoulder and then drop your right ear to your right shoulder. You may need to adjust the angle of your head to find the stretch in the left side of your neck. Once you have found the stretch stay here for 5-10 breaths. Gently place your right hand to the right side of your face to carefully lift your head back to centre. Repeat on the opposite side.

Breathing:

Coloured Breath: Close your eyes and notice if there is any tension in your body. Now imagine your breath as a colour. It can be any colour – there's no significance. As you breathe deeply, begin to send this colour to any part of your body which needs to relax. I imagine my breath is coloured smoke. There may be many parts of your body stressed, but do each one in turn.

Meditation:

Body Scan: Find a comfortable position, this may be seated or laying down and close your eyes. Starting from your toes, become aware of each body part in turn; feet, ankles, calves, knees, etc. all the way up to your head. Acknowledge the sensations you can feel in each body part. This technique can really help when trying to fall asleep.

Chapter 15: The Long Night

It was dark in the ward as I sat on the bed. There were 5 beds in total in my room. All had the curtains drawn. The sounds of beeping machines cut through the air. Suddenly I was hungry so I dug into the stash of food my parents had brought in. I felt my chest, it was icy cold.

I went to the toilet to take another peek and the bruising on my nipples seemed worse. They didn't look good. I asked the nurse for her opinion and, concerned, she called for the duty doctor. I'm not sure how long I waited for him to show up but it felt like forever.

He examined me and told me that it was touch and go. We just needed to wait and see if the circulation would return to my nipples. It was much too early to say. Apparently, the best thing for me to do was go to bed and rest. I felt queasy as I struggled to put my hospital gown back on.

It's a funny thing, when a doctor or nurse examines you they help you out of the gown. Once they have seen you they go, leaving you to dress yourself. I couldn't reach very far back so this was a real struggle. Over the next two days this happened a lot!

I couldn't just rest. I knew I had to help my circulation, so I devised a plan. A plan to keep my nipples. I was going to do everything possible and I knew lying in bed wouldn't help me at all. I realised I needed to keep drinking water to flush out all the medicine which had been pumped into me and keep moving to help my circulation. I also had to keep my chest warm and above all else keep a positive mindset. Once I had a plan I felt stronger.

I asked the nurse for a hot water bottle which I wrapped in a blanket and held against my chest. The whole area was completely numb in some places and horrendously painful in others as the painkillers were starting to wear off. The nurses were run off their feet, so I filled a few jugs of water. I untangled the drip, straightened my drains and refastened them to the stand so I was more mobile. By this time, it was after 2am and I was exhausted but I had to keep going. I was now ready to start my routine.

Firstly, I drank 2 cups of water. I then did some simple neck, arm and leg exercises by the side of my bed. These lasted for about 5 minutes. Next, I walked out of the room and along the corridor 4 times. I walked slowly and tried to breathe deeply. I then walked back to my bed to start the whole thing again. The routine lasted about 15 minutes. Every second or third round I needed the toilet. I also got some fresh hot water bottles during the night. In the end the nurses were fed up trying to get me to go to bed so they left me to it.

I was uncomfortable and tired. The hot water bottle was heavy in my arms and pushing the drip stand was awkward, but I knew I had to keep going.

After the first 2 hours I looked again at my nipples. To me they looked a tiny bit better but I'm not sure if that's just what I wanted to see. It was all the encouragement I needed to continue with the routine. Drinking, stretching, walking….drinking, stretching, walking…again and again and again. I'm not sure why but it didn't occur to me to put my headphones on. I suppose I just wanted the silence. I was using all my knowledge of anatomy and just sheer gut instinct to give myself the best possible chance.

By 7am I was sure that my nipples weren't quite as shrivelled. I was completely shattered. I sat in the chair by my bed and closed my eyes. I awoke a short while later to the clatter of breakfast. I hungrily ate some toast.

Then the drugs trolley came round. They wanted to give me painkillers but I didn't want them. I hadn't taken any since just after the operation. I was in pain but I could bear it. I needed to feel what was happening in my body as opposed to it being numb. I also knew that the quickest way out of the hospital was to not take the painkillers, so the doctors would think I was okay to go home. This was my goal and what I wanted more than anything... just to go home.

Refusing pain relief meant they took the cannula out, so now I could lose the stand and I just had my drains in a bag. There was hardly any fluid in the drains, slightly more in the left side. By the time Mr H came to examine me, I had washed myself the best I could and had even done some gentle yoga by my bed which included sitting on a spare sheet on the floor. The other patients in the ward must have thought I was mad!

Mr H told me that the left side had been really tricky as the skin was so thin. They wanted to remove as much of the breast tissue as possible so they had to go as close to the skin as they could. As well as the stitches underneath both breasts I also had further stitches at the top of my left breast and in my cleavage on the right side.

Mr H said that my nipples would probably survive but during the next few weeks we would know more. He was concerned about the area of skin underneath my left nipple. The skin here had been damaged and it looked like I had been burnt. It was oozy and angry looking. Mr H said that if it didn't heal then he needed to think about skin grafts. For now I had to keep a dressing on that area.

I told him I wanted to go home today, but he said that I needed to be in for at least another night. He also urged me to take the pain relief but I refused. I thanked him for making sure my operation went ahead and he told me not to thank him yet as we had a long way to go. This didn't sound like good news.

Next I had a visit from the physio. She was very surprised to see me up and about. She told me that she would help me to walk up the corridor. Yes, the same corridor that I'd walked up and down all night. I knew I probably needed a 'tick' from her to get discharged so I humoured her. After our walk she went through the exercises she had given me in a booklet. I had already completed all of them and more. They were extremely basic.

Luckily I didn't have cancer, so I realise that for somebody who did and had my type of operation, their mobility might be very different. For someone like me though who was fit and active the exercises were far too easy. I knew that I had to continue to use my intuition to know which movements were right for my body. I would have to rehabilitate myself.

My parents and Steven were on their way so I decided to sneak out the hospital and wait for them by the front door. I needed the fresh air. I could see from the window that it was a beautiful sunny autumn day. I decided to make a run for it.

Armed with my drains and an extra blanket I crept past the nurses and into the lift. It was crowded and I worried that I would be pushed. The thought of someone's elbow knocking into my new breasts was too much to bear. Once out of the lift I walked to freedom. Even though I had only been in the hospital about 30 hours at that point it seemed like a lifetime. As I gulped in the crisp air I instantly felt better. It was a little cold so I put the blanket around me and sat in the sunniest spot I could find.

I thought that my parents and Steven would be there any minute, but in fact it took them nearly half an hour. They had entered the hospital through the back door and gone up to my ward. The nurses had told them I had stepped outside (they must have seen me after all!) and they eventually came to the front of the hospital to find me.

I could see how relieved they were to see me up and about. My Dad had brought me some soup and we sat outside whilst I ate it. I skimmed over the events of the previous night as I didn't want them to worry too much, but I did tell them what Mr H had said.

The rest of the day passed slowly, all sitting around my bed. Time was only punctuated with the nurses doing my obs and changing my dressings. I was so restless and I just wanted to go home. Steven and I spent most of the day walking up and down the corridor. I also sat on his lap a lot as it was the only way we could cuddle.

In the evening a friend came to visit me. She brought me a goody bag with lovely herbal teas and an adult colouring book. She told me I looked good and couldn't believe I'd had a major operation the previous day. As the five of us sat there chatting, I prepared myself for another night trapped in the hospital.

Yoga For Survival

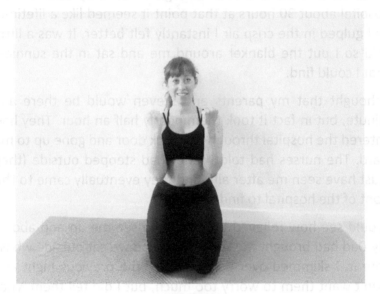

Bicep Curl

Poses:

The poses I did during my long night are as follows. The neck, hand and arm poses can be performed seated or standing.

Neck Release: (Chapter 14)

Hand Stars: Begin with your fist clenched. Breathing continuously, stretch your hands wide and then close them into fists. Repeat 20 times.

Bicep Curl: Begin with your arms by your sides with your palms facing up. Inhale and slowly bend your elbows so that your hands come up towards your shoulders. As you do this clench your fists. Exhale, uncurl your fists and release your arms by the side of your body. Repeat 5 times.

Arm Lift: Begin with your arms by your sides. Inhale lift arms in front of you up to shoulder height, exhale lower arms back down. Repeat 5 times. You can also repeat this movement extending your arms to the side shoulder height. After my operation I couldn't lift my arms to shoulder height, but I worked towards this target for a week or two.

Knee Raises: Begin in the standing position (Chapter 8). If you are unsteady you can hold on to the wall. Inhale, lift knee so it is in line with your hip, exhale release foot to floor. 10 times on each side.

Heel to Butt: Begin in the standing position (Chapter 8). If you are unsteady you can hold on to the wall. Inhale, kick foot behind you as close to your bottom as possible, exhale release foot to floor. 10 times on each side.

Breathing:

Magic Hands: Place your hands on your injured area and close your eyes. Breathe in and out calmly through your nose. Feel the heat of your hands and begin to direct your breath to this area. Know you have the ability to heal yourself. Stay here for as long as feels good.

Meditation:

Walking Meditation: (Chapter 8). As I roamed around the corridors, I tried to concentrate on each step I took. This really focussed my mind.

Chapter 16: Heal Thy Self

As soon as my visitors had left a new patient arrived on the ward. The previous lady next to me had left earlier that day. She had been in over a week as she had breast cancer and a breast reconstruction from her belly. She was dreading going home and really wanted to stay in for longer but they needed the bed.

This seemed to be a common theme in the ward. The women just wanted to stay. They also treated the drugs like sweets and took as many as they were offered. Now I'm not saying that they weren't in pain, but how would they know as they had been taking painkillers continuously for weeks.

Pain isn't pleasant but if you can't feel anything then how do you know when you are healing? These ladies also weren't prepared to do anything for themselves and called the nurses at any opportunity. I overheard the physio telling one of them that they were perfectly okay to use the toilet unaided. When the physio had gone the first thing the patient did was to call the nurse to take her to the toilet!

I truly believe that you have to help yourself. You cannot rely on the medical professionals, you need to make the effort to rehabilitate yourself. Of course, rest is vital, but I believe movement and deep breathing are important too.

Although the ladies in the ward moaned constantly about the nurses (often to their faces), I thought they did a great job. Often overworked and under staffed I could really see they were doing their best. I was always polite and friendly towards them. As a result, they were friendly and chatty to me. The main nurse who looked after me enjoyed telling me about her son who was at university studying to be a doctor. I liked this chit chat as it took me out of my own troubled thoughts.

Apart from talking to the nurses, I didn't really speak to the other patients. The ladies were either moaning or watching TV. I greatly believe that you need to surround yourself with positive people to feel better and the air of negativity seemed to hang in the air. On the few occasions I made conversation I tried to jolly them along, but they were unresponsive.

The lady in the bed next to me looked a very scary sight. I had no idea what was wrong with her but her whole face was bandaged. She was plugged in to countless machines and she was crying and screaming. I wasn't planning to sleep that night as I had to keep my circulation going, but sleep wasn't an option anyway.

Later, as I went about my routine the cries of the mummified lady rang out all over the ward. One nurse stayed with her all night and others came to check on her too. Fed up with trying to get me to go to bed, the nurses left me alone. Some of them told me that it was so refreshing to see someone trying so hard to recover. I didn't know if I was doing the right thing, but it felt right to me.

My nipples had begun to look a bit better so maybe my plan was working. At around 5am I got a few hours' sleep sitting upright in the chair. When I woke up I did some gentle yoga and washed. Body wipes were my saving grace and made such a difference. By the time Mr H came to check on me in the morning I was sitting at the table, colouring the book my friend had given me. It was a Halloween pattern.

After examining me and realising that I hadn't taken even one painkiller since my operation, he said that I could go home that day. On average patients stay in 5 nights but I couldn't handle another night. He also thought my nipples were looking slightly better. I needed to leave with my drains then return to the hospital in four days' time to have them removed. I was going home!

After the breast care nurse had fitted me with a sports bra for support, I nagged the nurses to get my discharge letter so I would be ready to leave. I knew this could take ages, so I pushed them to chase it. I wanted to be out of the hospital by lunchtime. When my Dad and Steven came to the hospital my bag was packed and I was ready.

After 50 long hours of being in hospital I stepped out in to the cool autumn air. As Hospital B is in north London and I live in south London, the quickest way to get back was by tube. I enjoyed the walk to the station carrying my drains. Blood was visible through the tubes, so it's lucky it was coming up to Halloween. I was dressed for it!

My Dad and Steven acted as bodyguards on the tube to make sure I wasn't pushed. It was great to be out of the hospital. I felt so alive. I was hugely relieved that I no longer had the scary percentages of getting cancer. Now I just needed to recover.

Yoga To Aid Healing

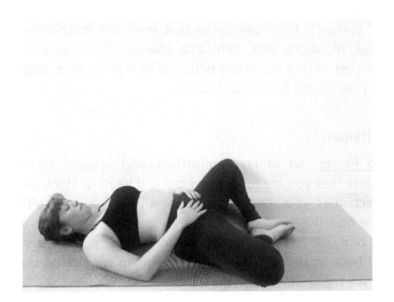

Supine Butterfly

Pose:

I continued with the poses in Chapter 15 and I also needed to release my hips. There is a lot of emotional tension caught up in this area, so this felt great.

Supine Butterfly: Lay on the floor or your bed and bring the soles of your feet together and let your knees drop open. You can use cushions or blocks to support your knees if required. Place your hands on your belly and breathe deeply. Stay until your hips and lower back release.

Breathing:

Peaceful Breath: Close your eyes and breathe steadily. Link the following phrase with your breath: 'This too' (inhale) 'shall pass' (exhale). This reminds us that even the most difficult, painful situations will shift and change. You can choose whichever phrase resonates with you at a given time. Repeat until your breath is even and steady.

Meditation:

Mind Power: Sit or lay comfortably and breathe steadily. Visualise that you are fully recovered and healthy. Think about the activities you are doing and the places you are visiting. Notice how this feels and gently breathe these sensations into your body. If you get distracted don't worry, just bring your mind back to the recovered you. The mind is more powerful than we know. Stay here for 5-10 minutes.

Chapter 17: Beginning To Heal

Back safely in my apartment, my Dad took over nursing duties. My drains kept leaking so the dressings needed to be changed every few hours. It was very uncomfortable when the wet dressings were against my skin. I developed a rash down both sides of my body and was constantly itchy. No fluid seemed to be collecting in my drains which was good. I lived in Steven's T-shirts as they were the only thing I could get over the drains.

As soon as I got home I was desperate for a shower and I needed to wash my hair. I couldn't get my dressings wet so I used a bin liner and made holes for my head and arms. Once this was on I tied it in a knot under my breasts. This allowed me to step into the shower cubicle and use the hand-held shower to wash my lower body.

This was part one of the process. Part two involved stepping out of the cubicle and drying my lower body. I then knelt on the mat and faced the cubicle, tipping my head forward. Steven held the shower over me so I could wash my hair. Although I couldn't lift my arms over my head, I managed to wash my hair keeping my elbows drawn into my ribs. The final part of the process involved taking the bin liner off and using body wipes to clean my underarms and my back.

This whole tedious mission took about 40 minutes. After the first time with Steven helping me I realised I could do it myself, I just needed him to pass me the shower head. I was even able to dry my own hair. There's nothing worse than someone helping you wash and dress. This actually makes you feel sick and I wasn't sick, I was recovering.

This whole situation is very strange. It's elective surgery, it's a choice. In a way you feel like a bit of a fraud. There are plenty of people with cancer having life-saving operations every day. I had put myself in this position but I didn't feel like I had any other choice.

In the days that followed life moved slowly with the drains. I kept forgetting to pick them up when I stood up and they dragged along the floor. They were also very uncomfortable. The worst thing however was having to sleep on my back. I was terrified I would turn on my side and disturb the drains. Also, if I laid on my side I would probably damage the reconstruction. I didn't want to end up back in surgery.

Even at my most unattractive with drains coming out of me, Steven and I were still intimate. I think that it's important to try and carry on as normal. I missed being able to cuddle properly, this was a long way off yet, but we did the best we could.

Every morning I made sure I rolled my yoga mat out and did what I could manage. I created modified versions of the sun salutations and enjoyed the challenge of adapting poses. I also realised I was getting stronger and had more movement each day. These daily practices kept me calm and grounded and I'm not sure what I would have done without them.

Previously I had taught some senior yoga classes. Although I adapted the poses to suit the class I didn't have any personal understanding of having limited movement. Now I understood. I was sure this experience was going to make me a better and more creative teacher.

I also started other gentle exercise. Steven and I owned a step and some weights. As we exercised together, I stepped up and down slowly and with the lightest weights. I must have looked a sight doing this with my drains! More than anything I just wanted to feel normal.

It took 3 days after surgery for anyone from Studio 666 to contact me. Then it was just a quick courtesy text. I knew they didn't care about me but this did surprise me. It was like they had no feelings at all. In contrast, from friends and family I received flowers, chocolates and lots of cards. I felt very spoilt.

Armed with chocolates for the nurses on the ward I had stayed in, Steven, my Mum and I made our way to Hospital B for the removal of my drains. I couldn't wait – I was so fed up dragging them around and the constant leaking. I had been told it hurt so I prepared myself.

We waited in the hot, overcrowded waiting room for nearly two hours. We busied ourselves by playing blackjack on my phone. Eventually I was called in. Steven came in the room with me and as I lay on the bed I held his hand. Firstly, the nurses removed the large plaster strip that were holding the implants down. This was a relief as I was hot and sticky underneath. For the first time I could see my new breasts and they looked great. Obviously, they were bruised and swollen but they looked good. I'd had no idea what I would be left with, but I had nipples and nicely shaped breasts.

Next came the removal of the drains. Steven squeezed my hand tighter. I thought that the drains were just inserted to the side of my breasts but in fact they reached all the way to underneath my nipples. I can't explain the feeling as the drains were removed but I wish they had done them both at the same time as after the first side, knowing I had to go through this again was horrible. I just tried to breathe as deeply as I could and imagine myself on a beach far away. The plan was that after I recovered, we would go on an amazing holiday, so each step I took felt as though I was getting closer to that point.

The skin under my left breast was still a concern. I didn't see Mr H that day but I did see one of his registrars. They said that the best way to treat the wound was with a manuka honey dressing. This seemed very new age to me but it smelt amazing. They gave me some to take home and I was told to redress it every day.

With the drains removed I was much more comfortable and mobile. I still couldn't get the area wet for a few weeks yet and I had to sleep on my back for a while longer, but it felt as though I was on the road to recovery.

Yoga To Support Healing

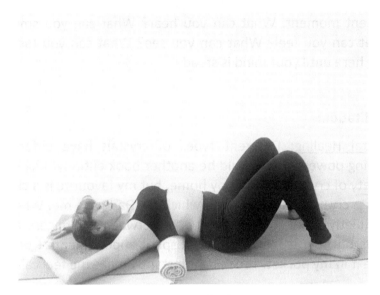

Lay Over Blanket

Pose:

After surgery the whole of my upper back seized up and was very tender. I found the following restorative pose very helpful.

Lay Over Blanket: Roll up a medium sized blanket and place it across your mat. Your aim is to lay over it on your back, so the blanket is just below your shoulder blades. You may need to adjust and if it feels too intense then use a thinner blanket. When you are comfortable, close your eyes and breathe deeply into your chest. This can also be performed with Legs Up The Wall (Chapter 2). Stay here for at least 5 minutes.

Breathing:

Mindful Breath: Sit or lay comfortably and breathe deeply in and out through your nose. Begin to fill your mind with the present moment. What can you hear? What can you smell? What can you feel? What can you see? What can you taste? Stay here until your mind is steady.

Meditation:

Crystal Healing: Different types of crystals have different healing powers – this could be another book entirely! I have a variety of crystals around my home, but my favourite is a clear quartz crystal shaped buddha which my Dad gave me. When I sit quietly I like to rub the crystal between my fingers and focus on how it feels. During hospital appointments I often have it in my pocket. Touching it instantly make me feel calm.

Chapter 18: Getting Stronger

When I had my ovaries and fallopian removed I didn't take any time off work. I stopped teaching my classes for a week, but I did my admin work for Studio 666 from home. This suited me as I wanted to keep the studio running as smoothly as possible. Nobody else would spend hours finding the appropriate cover for classes when the regular teachers were unable to teach. I took pride in my job and wanted the classes, workshops and teachers' trainings to be the best possible.

Even though I completed my hours, my mean boss deducted a week's wages from my pay cheque. I couldn't believe that after working so hard straight after my first operation she would do this to me but she did. I didn't confront her about this but was deeply hurt.

This time round I had learned my lesson. After my breast operation I booked a week off work (unpaid!) and didn't check my emails once. Shortly before the week was up a staff member contacted me and asked for my address. She told me that my boss 'thought that she should send flowers' and they wanted to check my address. When the bouquet arrived, I saw it as an afterthought and something they felt they had to do so it didn't mean anything.

For the first few weeks after surgery I went to see my healer every week. She was fantastic. I felt amazing after each session and it was great to be able to talk to someone outside my family and friends. Although I was still sore, bruised and struggling to sleep on my back, I always slept more peacefully after the sessions.

When I showered and changed my dressings daily I had a chance to look at myself in the mirror. This was hard to do. As well as my still visible scars on my belly from my first surgery, my new breasts were bruised and scarred. The skin on my left breast looked like something out of a horror film. A scab was slowly forming which the hospital told me meant the skin underneath was healing.

I've always thought that I didn't place a huge amount of importance on appearance, that what's inside counts for more. This whole process really tested this belief. Could I still feel attractive with my new breasts? How was I going to look at the end? The shape was good now but would it change? So many questions floated around when I looked in the mirror. Some days I didn't want to look but I forced myself. I needed to recognise that this was me.

I also knew that I was far luckier than others – burn victims, amputees for example – I had it easy. But this was my body, my experience, so I had to let myself go through all the emotions. I knew this was part of the healing process. It was okay that I often felt out of my depth and teary when I saw my reflection.

I made the effort to dress nicely and took time with my hair and make-up. This made me feel a little better. Although sex was tricky as no pressure could be put on my chest, I still felt confident. I had to wear a sports bra day and night to support my breasts so with this on I didn't look any different. I allowed Steven to see my wounds when I changed my dressing and he continually told me that the shape was good and once everything healed, I would look great. I struggled to believe him as I felt sore in some places, numb in others but I hoped he was right.

Two weeks after surgery I went back to teaching. Previously I had been teaching some classes in the hot room, but I knew this was out of bounds as I had open wounds and there was risk of infection. I was getting stronger each day in my own practice so I knew I could teach a class. I wouldn't be able to demonstrate all the poses but I could call on good students to do this for me.

My first class back was a really gentle floor based class. My Dad came to the class and it was lovely to have the support. I hadn't told any of the students at Studio 666 about my operations as I didn't want to be bombarded with questions. I'm not good at dealing with sympathy. My boss sent another staff member into the class to spy on me as she was worried that I would sue if anything happened to me after surgery. It was my choice to go back as I wanted to get back to normality. I was taking the risks but I knew my body well enough to know I was strong enough. Rather than my boss asking how I was feeling, as usual she was just concerned about herself.

It was nice to get back to some sort of routine. I was gently exercising and eating well. One Friday, three and a half weeks after surgery, I noticed that my left nipple had turned a pale colour and was really shrivelled. It didn't look good. In a panic I called the emergency line to the hospital. They said I could come in first thing in the morning, otherwise it would be a long wait in A&E. I decided to go for the first option.

I was in a real state, I even went through the embarrassment of showing my Dad. He thinks of himself as a bit of a doctor. He said that if the circulation had stopped completely then the skin would have turned black. I spent the evening watching mindless TV, with a hot bottle over my chest, trying not to think about what could happen tomorrow.

My Mum and I waited most of the next morning to be seen. I thought the nipple looked slightly pinker but I couldn't be sure. As the registrar examined me, I tried to steady my breath. He told me that the skin of the nipple had become dry and flaky, but it was absolutely fine. He even flaked a bit of skin off to show me the pink skin underneath.

What a relief! If only someone had told me that this could happen I would have been prepared. I know they can't tell you about every eventuality, but I hadn't slept at all the previous night, scared that I would be rushed into surgery the next morning and they would have to remove my nipple.

As the next few weeks passed I neared the end of the nipple danger zone and it appeared they were there to stay. The wound under my left nipple had formed a hard scab. This was still being treated with the manuka honey dressing which I was told would eventually loosen the scab. It all looked good. I was recovering.

Yoga To Build Strength

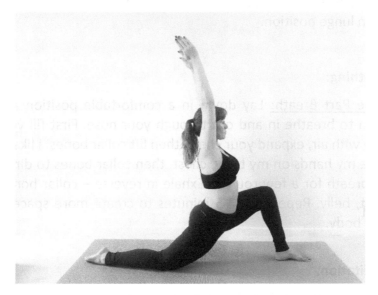

Lunge

Pose:

Lunge: Lunges release tension in the lower back whilst opening the front of the hips and thighs. Start on hands and knees. Perform some cat/cow stretches (Chapter 6). Then gently step your left foot between your hands so that your knee is stacked over your ankle. For a deeper stretch you can move your right knee back a few inches. Try to square your hips by rolling your right hip forward. If your hands do not reach the floor you can use blocks. To progress, gently tuck your bottom under and reach your arms overhead with your palms facing and your shoulders relaxed. Stay here for 5 breaths. To come out of the pose, place your hands on the floor or blocks so you can bring your left knee to meet your right knee. Repeat on the right side.

During recovery I also practiced the arm exercises (Chapter 15) in lunge position.

Breathing:

<u>Three Part Breath:</u> Lay down in a comfortable position and begin to breathe in and out through your nose. First fill your belly with air, expand your chest, then lift collar bones. I like to place my hands on my belly, chest, then collar bones to direct my breath for a few rounds. Exhale in reverse – collar bones, chest, belly. Repeat for 2-5 minutes to create more space in your body.

Meditation:

<u>Taste Meditation</u>: My Mum introduced me to Rescue Remedy Pastilles and I have come to rely on them to soothe me. I like to sit quietly and notice the sensation of the pastille in my mouth. I notice the texture, flavour and how it begins to melt and coat my tongue. I always carry them with me for moments when I need to find tranquillity.

Chapter 19: Bad News

I was in less pain and I had more mobility. I was also able to do much more in my yoga practice. I constantly had a strange feeling on the inside edge of my left shoulder blade. It felt achy but also numb and damp. During sessions with my healer she also noticed there was a damp feeling on my left side. Although it didn't feel quite right I just put it down to the healing process.

On 8th December 2016, Steven and I went back to Hospital B for an appointment with Mr H. We thought he would be pleased with my progress and allow me to move from these weekly trips to less frequent appointments.

I was examined by a doctor who I hadn't seen before. By now I had been seen by just about every nurse and doctor in the clinic, but this doctor was new to me. She had a very stern manner and when Steven asked if we would be seeing Mr H she seemed very offended. After examination, she said they would remove the scab today on my left breast. I was thrilled. It felt like this was the last hurdle to get over.

The registrar and the nurse began to lay everything out ready for the removal of my scab. It was about an inch square and was strangely in the rough shape of a heart. I was excited at the thought of seeing my left breast without it. I held on to Steven's hand as the registrar bent over me. As she begun to lift the scab away from the skin she stopped. She said that she would be back in a minute. I just thought she had to go to the toilet.

She returned with Mr H. Steven quickly began to thank him and tell him that he had done a great job. In his usual matter-of-fact tone, Mr H told him not to thank him yet as there could be a problem. I went cold. Mr H had a look at the scab and I could see the concern in his eyes. The skin had not grown back underneath as hoped. There was a large hole in the skin of my left breast. I had been very lucky not to get an infection.

I asked Mr H if it was due to anything I had done – maybe I should have rested more? He assured me that this wasn't the case – sometimes the skin just doesn't heal. The reconstruction involved making a bra of pigskin which lay underneath my skin. This made the structure strong enough to support the implant. Underneath the scab the implant was visible.

As Mr H told me they would need to operate on me the next morning the room began to spin. This was an emergency. Mr H needed to completely remove the implant on my left side, stitch up the hole and allow the skin to heal. A temporary implant would be inserted and gradually inflated over time once the skin had knitted. I didn't know how long I would be without a left breast.

I felt numb and wanted to cry at the same time. I thought I was healing. I thought I was fine. I could tell Mr H was troubled and he could tell I was frightened. He told me not to worry and that it would be all right. As much as I trusted him and his skill I just didn't know what to think.

Somewhere in the middle of all this trauma, I found out that no sign of cancer had been detected in my breast tissue. We should have been celebrating instead we left the hospital in a state of shock. Another operation. Tomorrow.

I called my parents and they couldn't believe it either. Up until now another operation hadn't even been mentioned but I was going to have one tomorrow. I couldn't face the tube journey just yet so we went to the local coffee shop. I've spent a lot of time here pre or post appointments. I'm a sucker for hot chocolate.

As it all sank in I began to cry. Not loud crying, just the type of crying when you really don't have any energy and tears just roll down your face. Steven held me close but he just didn't know what to say. There's nothing anyone could say. It was just devastating.

As thoughts went through my mind of only having one breast, the practical, organised part of me kicked in too. I needed to tell work, get my classes covered and I was supposed to be going to the theatre with my friend the following evening. Steven was booked on a train in an hour's time, as he had work that weekend in Leeds.

He said he would wouldn't go home but that made me feel very awkward. I didn't want him to miss out on work. I only wanted him to stay if he felt that he couldn't possibly be anywhere else, not out of a sense of duty.

As he spoke to his parents and told them about the past few hours' events his Mum told him that of course he must stay. His Dad on the other hand had the opposing opinion and told him to come back for work. I overheard the whole conversation. I know his Dad was just looking out for him, but it came across so clearly that the only thing he thought about was money. This made the whole situation worse and made me even more upset. I know that his Dad didn't mean to upset me, that it is just his way, but nevertheless it hurt. I have since forgiven him (in my own mind), but I will never forget.

In the end Steven decided to stay with me. Once back at home, we set about putting our lives on hold again for yet another operation. Within a few hours everything was either cancelled or rescheduled. My hospital bag was packed. I wondered how this had happened.

Yoga For Coping With Bad News

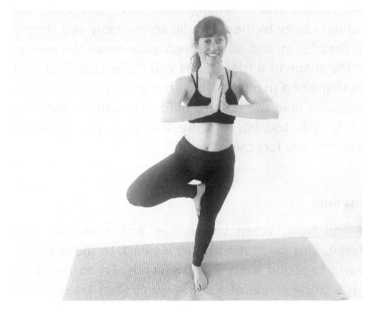

Tree

Pose:

Tree: This pose brings mental clarity and focusses the mind. Begin in a steady standing position (Chapter 8). Find a focus point along the floor and softly fix your gaze there. Gently turn out your left hip and place the sole of the left foot on the inside of your right leg. You can place the foot on your ankle, calf or higher up the leg on your thigh, depending on your flexibility (anywhere but the knee). As you press your foot into your leg bring your hands to prayer position. Stay here for 5 breaths. Repeat on the right side.

Breathing:

Triangle Breath: When we are completely overwhelmed we become tense. This breathing exercise regulates the breath and brings clarity to the mind. Sit comfortably and close your eyes. Breathe in and out through your nose. On your palm trace the shape of a triangle. As you move your finger slowly in the shape of a triangle match your breath. First side: inhale; second side: hold the breath; third side: exhale. Don't worry about breath counts, just breathe with your movement. Repeat until you feel calm.

Meditation:

Here and Now: When we receive bad news our mind is scattered. This meditation brings us back to the present. Set an alarm to sound every 20-30 seconds. Try to find a sound that is a single chime of a bell. As you sit or lay comfortably with steady breath, begin to clear your mind. Every time you hear the chime it will instantly bring you back to the present moment. Use these chimes as a reminder that we can only live in the present and not get caught up in 'what ifs'. Repeat for 2-5 minutes.

Chapter 20: Staying Positive

Once again we checked in at the hospital at 7:30am but this time my wait was not as long or as turbulent. Mr H was keen to get me into theatre. The longer the hole was there, I was at more risk of infection. I could end up with no left breast if that happened.

In a way I'm pleased this operation happened so quickly. I didn't have much time to think about the fact that when I woke up from surgery I would be flat on my left side. As Steven, my parents and I sat in the waiting corridor, my left side began to ache. It's like it knew it was about to be disturbed again. It made sense now why I felt dampness in my left shoulder blade. It hadn't healed.

I was a pro at this now, so I padded down to surgery armed again with a pillow. I didn't feel as anxious. I looked forward to the pre-med so the thoughts dancing around my mind would disappear. I didn't know how I would feel or how I would look afterwards, but I just wanted it over.

I woke up to the now familiar sound of beeping machines. I didn't feel as groggy as the operation wasn't as long as the last one. The nurse made checks around me and I looked under the sheets at my chest. My left breast was flat, my right breast looked huge in comparison. I thought instantly of my Auntie. During her fight with breast cancer she had a single mastectomy. I wondered how she must have felt waking up. It must have been worse for her as she had cancer. I didn't, but I still looked down in disbelief at my flat left side. I consoled myself that at least I didn't have drains this time.

One of Mr H's registrars checked me over and told me they had been able to repair the hole in my skin. I wouldn't need a skin graft which was a relief. The plan was to let the skin heal then inflate the breast over time. I asked how long it would take and he said it was much too early to tell and that the main priority was that the skins heals. I would be uneven for a while it seemed. Sensing my disappointment, the nurse suggested that I use a filler in the left side of my bra. I knew I didn't want to do this – the world would just have to cope seeing me with uneven breasts.

I was moved quite quickly to the ward where my parents and Steven were waiting. They were obviously concerned but I said that I was okay, even if I wasn't sure that was the truth. The nurses told that I may need to stay in overnight but I was determined to go home. I got out of bed, supporting myself with my right hand and began to walk around.

Again I refused the painkillers and pushed for a release time. As my obs were good, after a few long hours of pacing around the corridor, it was agreed that I could leave. I locked the door of the toilet and began to take off my hospital gown. I didn't want to look at my body but I forced myself. This was me after all, I needed to face what I looked like now.

It was an odd sight. My right breast sat there all perky and evenly shaped, but my left breast was like a deflated balloon. It looked like it had been dehydrated. The nipple was still intact which was something to be thankful for. A large white plaster covered the bottom of my breast so I couldn't see the scar. This was attached to a tube and a small box. The nurse told me that this box would help to keep the moisture away from the area.

Once my bra was on, I stared at the empty left side where my breast should have been. Luckily at 32C my breasts weren't that big, but when I was dressed the difference was noticeable. I quickly put on my baggy jumper and we left the hospital.

Once outside in the cold winter air, I felt strangely euphoric. And brave. Maybe it was the medication or just sheer relief that I was out of the hospital as I haven't thought of myself as brave before or since. I was proud that even though one of my worst nightmares had been realised I was still here, still standing. I actually felt good.

We were all starving so we went to have pizza. I even had a beer. I checked the leaflet that came with my antibiotics and it didn't mention alcohol so I took the chance. That hot, spicy pizza and cold beer seemed like the best meal I'd ever had.

I slept peacefully that night, even though I now had to return to sleeping on my back. I was in pain but it didn't compare to the first breast operation. I knew that I could get over this operation much quicker than the last. I was going to be fine.

Yoga For A Positive Mind

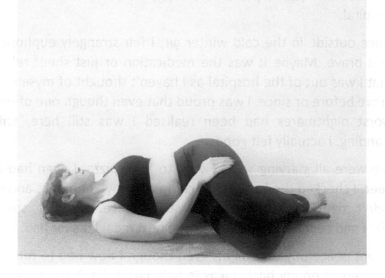

Supine Twist

Pose:

<u>Supine Twist</u>: Twists help to detoxify the body and mind. Lay on your mat comfortably with your knees bent and your feet flat on the floor. Shift your hips a few inches to the left and allow your knees to drop open to the right-hand side. If the knees don't come to the floor you can place a block or blanket between your thighs for support. Spread your arms wide. You can either look towards the ceiling or the opposite way to your knees. Begin to breathe deeply into the left-hand side of your rib cage. Feel this area expand deeply. Stay here for 2 minutes and then repeat on the other side.

Breathing:

Riding the Waves: Sit or lay comfortably and breathe in and out through your nose. Imagine that you are sitting on the beach watching the rolling waves. Begin to align your breath with the rhythm of the sea; inhale as the wave lifts and exhale as the water falls. Feel your breath become tranquil and steady. Repeat for 2 minutes.

Meditation:

Gratitude: It sounds strange, but even in the most difficult situations there are always many things to be grateful for. When you wake up instead of reaching for your phone and getting bogged down with the day's events, give yourself a few minutes to breathe and list the people/things you cherish. Your day will begin in a better place, whatever your situation.

Chapter 21: Dark Days

I woke up the next morning with a heavy heart. It was like the world had come crashing down around me. I grabbed my yoga mat, maybe exercise would make me feel better. I tried my best to breathe and move. I mentally listed all the good things in my life. This helped slightly, but I just felt so depleted. Then I started to cry and I couldn't stop.

Steven tried to comfort me, but I couldn't put into words how I was feeling. I was confused. Confused and very uneven. My right side was nearly back to normal but my left side was sore and weak. When I looked down at my chest I cried even more. I'll never forget having a shower that morning, I couldn't bear to look at myself in the mirror. I was back once again to showering in bin liners – I'd only just got away from that!

We walked, watched films, took gentle exercise but it was no good. I just felt dreadful. My parents knew how bad I felt and they tried to jolly me along but they must have been worried.

I've never been a person to be down, but the days after this operation I didn't know how to pick myself up. I think it was the complete shock of what had happened. One minute I was healing well and the next I had another surgery and I was back to square one. Now I had further surgery ahead of me. I had wanted to get it all over by the end of 2016. I was just so disappointed.

I was also very uncomfortable. The dressing was so itchy. Eventually I removed the itchy plaster that covered my left breast as I couldn't stand it anymore.

When my friend called I explained how awful I felt. She thought this was completely understandable and I should just give myself some time and space to allow it all to sink in. She reminded me that I always expect things to happen quickly and after going through so much, I probably just needed some time to adjust.

This conversation helped me. I realised I needed to look after myself and allow everything to settle. I also carried with me some guilt. After all I was lucky – I could do something to hopefully prevent cancer. There are many women, including many in my family, who didn't have that luxury – they just got cancer. There was a side of me that thought I should appreciate my circumstances and feeling low was disrespectful to them. I saw my healer a lot during this time.

Three days after surgery I woke up and my left breast had grown back! It was pretty much completely flat following surgery and now it filled the bra cup again. It didn't look swollen, it just looked how it did pre-surgery. I was overjoyed. I looked the same again! It was like a miracle.

My joy was short-lived as I realised this could perhaps be an infection or another problem. After a frantic call to the hospital they told me to come straight in. I saw a duty doctor who could not find any signs of infection and told me that I was healing well. I still had an uneasy feeling but knowing that I had an appointment with Mr H the following week put my mind at rest.

Gradually, I began to feel more like myself and I started to look ahead. It was only two weeks until Christmas. Steven, my Dad and I put up a new Christmas tree in my apartment. It looked beautiful and I hoped that by the time the tree went up next year all of this would be over.

After a 2 hour wait to see Mr H the following week, the look on his face told me I had been right to be concerned about my 'miracle' breast. It was fluid which might disperse naturally but if it didn't then it would have to be syringed. This procedure was not dangerous but it did mean an increased risk of infection which could be very serious. It was going to be a waiting game.

For my birthday Steven had booked a week away in Lanzarote. It didn't seem as though we would be able to go because I wouldn't be able to travel with this amount of fluid. We were so disappointed. We desperately needed a break.

Luckily after a few more trips to see Mr H, he was satisfied I was okay to travel. He had to write me a letter stating that I had metal in my temporary implant which may activate the metal detectors at the airport. The implant was very strange. There was quite a large piece of metal at the top of it which is where they would inflate it from. Feeling a piece of metal in your breast is very odd.

We managed to escape in the second week of January 2017. Unfortunately it wasn't sunny and we both got the flu as soon as we got off the plane. I think the months of stress and uncertainty all came rushing out when we had the chance to relax. Even so we had a great time, eating good food, listening to live music and walking along the beach. I even wore a bikini for a few hours.

I knew that on my return I would begin the process of having my left breast inflated. The skin had healed well. Mr H had done a fantastic job repairing the hole and the skin lay flat and neat. He was pleased with the result and I could tell it was a good outcome.

The first time Mr H inflated my left breast I didn't know what to expect. The nurse laid out various instruments of torture so I got the impression it would hurt. As Steven held my hand, I looked at the syringe which held saline. This was to be inserted through the metal plate into the temporary implant. This was ironic. I had waited weeks for the fluid to leave but now they were actually going to inject fluid back in. I couldn't help but feel sorry for my left side.

The plan was to inflate the breast slowly so not to disturb the skin that was still healing. When the breast was inflated back to its original size I would be ready for surgery to exchange the temporary implant.

The injection was a very strange sensation. The metal inside seemed to make this part of my skin extra sensitive. It felt like the needle was moving through very delicate tissue and instantly the breast started to inflate. It was just like a balloon. The pain was intense, but thankfully only lasted a matter of minutes. When you've been poked and prodded as much as I had at that point you get very used to managing pain. I had 6 injections in total over a 3 month period.

This process had a huge effect on my left side. After each injection my arm and hand felt numb and tingly, not a nice sensation. This lasted for days. I also developed knots in my left shoulder and the whole area felt tight. My left shoulder blade felt fragile and painful. My healer explained this best by saying when she held my left shoulder blade it felt like 'a broken wing of a bird'. My left side was damaged and very weak.

Through yoga and exercise, I gradually began to rebuild my left side. It took time and a lot of patience. I went to the gym and began to swim which I always find meditative. The exercise was hard enough but the most challenging part was the changing rooms. Women just stared at me as I changed. Some even asked if I had been attacked. I felt extremely uncomfortable and very, very ugly. I left the leisure centre crying more than once.

I caught myself one day changing in the toilet before swimming. I've never done this before. I suddenly thought – why I am I hiding away? To make other people feel more comfortable? I went out and changed with everyone else. If everyone with less than perfect bodies hides, then we are just conforming to the media's depiction of normality. To hell with them.

Yoga To Aid Sleep

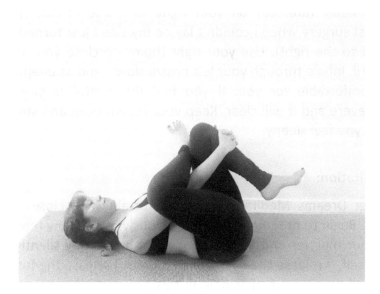

Supine Pigeon

Pose:

Supine Pigeon: This pose is great to release tension in the lower back and hips. This was fantastic during the time I had to sleep on my back. Lay on your back with your knees bent and your feet hip distance and parallel. Inhale, cross your right ankle over your left knee. Flex your right foot to protect your knee. Stay here for a few deep breaths. If this is enough of a stretch, then stay here. If you want to move deeper, lift your left foot away from the floor. Reach your hands through the gap either side of the left leg and around your hamstring or shin. If your hands cannot reach, then use a strap or a towel. Stay here for 10 breaths and then repeat on the other side. It feels good to move into a Supine Twist (Chapter 20) after this pose.

Breathing:

Sleepy Breath: This breath will help calm your mind and slow your heart rate. Lay on your right-hand side in bed (post breast surgery when I couldn't lay on my side I just turned my head to the right). Use your right thumb to close your right nostril. Inhale through your left nostril slowly and as deeply as is comfortable for you. If you find this nostril is blocked persevere and it will clear. Keep your breath even and steady until you feel sleepy.

Meditation:

Sweet Dreams Meditation: Lay comfortably and close your eyes. Begin to breathe deeply. Consciously release any tension in your muscles and let your body feel heavy. Say silently to yourself, 'I release the past and all regrets. I release the future and all worries. I reside only in this moment where I am at peace and free of all expectations.' Take a deep inhale and a slow exhale, consciously letting go of the past and the future. Visualise any negative energy, thoughts and feelings leaving your body. Sink into a deep, restful sleep.

Chapter 22: New Beginnings

By February 2017 my left breast was inflated fully. I hoped that during the summer I would have my (fingers crossed) final operation to exchange the implant.

After my first breast operation, we had a booked a holiday of a lifetime for March 2017, believing that everything was behind us. It was going to be a celebration that all the bad stuff was over, but unfortunately that was not to be.

Even though I had another operation pending, we had an incredible time. We visited Las Vegas, LA and took a cruise around the Hawaiian Islands. It was everything I had dreamt it would be and more. Just being so far away from home did me the world of good. Without the usual round of hospital appointments, I really relaxed.

I could never completely forget what had happened. The scars on my belly were still a little red and my left breast was sore. In the hot sun the metal inside seemed to heat up and became uncomfortable. Although I felt and looked a little uneven I wore a bikini and let the sun heal my body.

Hawaii is a very spiritual place, the volcanoes hold special powers. I allowed all this to wash over me and I began to feel renewed. Steven took some great photos of me doing yoga on the ship and in Hawaii to use on my website. Although I'd had a website for over a year, I hadn't really done anything with it. These pictures would kick start me into finishing it.

Two major life changes happened whilst we were away. On the third night of our holiday, whilst in Vegas, Steven proposed. We were sitting at the Blackjack table (our favourite vice) when he dropped to one knee and asked me to marry him. I'd had a lot of drinks that night so my memories are a little hazy but I said 'yes'. I honestly thought that he was joking.

Both of us had managed to avoid marriage and I thought we were happy that way. As we talked over the following days he explained that he wanted us to be together always and that's why we should get married. He felt it was important that he propose now rather than wait until after my final op. He wanted to be with me however I ended up looking.

Our living situation wouldn't change – my life in London, his in Leeds, but it was a way for us to be more connected. I wanted the same, so I slowly began to come around to the idea. I told him that if we could find a way to get married that felt like 'us' then it would be a lovely thing to do. After all, Steven had been with me through the most difficult time of my life.

I couldn't stand the thought of a big wedding with everyone watching me and having to invite people you don't really know and often don't really like. Our gut instinct was to go away just the two of us and get married, but we really wanted our parents to be there. In the end we decided that we wanted to get married on a cruise ship. We loved going on cruises and the idea felt like 'us'.

Before we told anyone back home I wanted Steven to ask my Dad. My Dad loves winding people up, so I knew he would have fun with Steven when he asked for his permission to marry me.

Although we were having a wonderful holiday I had a nagging feeling about my job. Studio 666 was becoming a very difficult place to work with my boss's mood swings. I still worked extremely hard and earnt my boss a lot of money but the job didn't make me happy. During the last meeting before I went away there was a strange atmosphere. It felt as though I had been left out of the loop. I kept telling Steven that I could feel something was happening, something was changing.

On my return, for a variety of reasons, my boss made it impossible for me to stay in my job so I resigned. Leaving also meant giving up most of my weekly classes as they were at Studio 666. I was left with no income.

Part of me felt relieved. I'd wanted to leave for a long time but felt trapped due to the job fitting in with my travel to Leeds. I knew I was underselling myself working there, but I didn't see another option until the end of my operations. Now I had to do something else.

I shed some tears and spent a few days feeling sorry for myself. When you return from a lovely holiday you always feel a bit out of sorts so I'm sure this didn't help. I carried on with the few classes I had left and put the feelers out for opportunities to pick up new classes. This didn't lead to much work, so I had no choice but to register for supply teaching.

Previously I had been a primary school teacher for 12 years. I enjoyed teaching children and loved the long summer holidays. I had left 4 years earlier to fully concentrate on personal training, group exercise and yoga. I felt that I had stopped school teaching at the right time. Although I enjoyed the teaching part, the paperwork was overwhelming and I didn't want to end up hating the job.

The idea of going back as a supply teacher was scary. I didn't know if I could still control a class. The schools in my area are tough and the kids eat supply teachers for breakfast. I needed to work so I just had to get on with it.

My first day back was terrifying. I got there early and studied the plans. The year 2 class were very lively and took no prisoners. When the bell rang and the kids came in, it was like I had never been away. I remembered all my 'tricks' for holding their attention and I actually quite liked the challenge of teaching them. It was a good day.

Unfortunately, not all my supply days were as good. I got jumped on and pushed to the ground by a big child with learning difficulties. I hurt my head and spent the rest of the day teaching with a splitting headache. Also as a supply teacher you are ignored by the regular teachers and they treat you as if you are stupid. Nobody speaks to you in the staffroom and it can be quite lonely. The teachers also give you all the lessons to cover that they don't want to teach. I taught a lot of PE and Art. I didn't mind as I like those subjects.

Once I was earning a small income, with my Dad's approval, we announced our engagement. Our parents were thrilled and our friends were shocked as nobody thought that either one of us would get married. People seemed to think it was strange as we obviously weren't going down the route of marriage then children, so I suppose they didn't see the point. All that mattered was it made sense to us.

We quickly booked our wedding on a week's cruise in the Mediterranean for June 2018. As we sipped champagne with my parents, I realised my life was changing rapidly. I felt very liberated and creative since I had left Studio 666. It was during this time that I began to write this book. Many people had commented how quickly I had recovered from my operations and they thought I should record this is some way.

I had recently read Elizabeth's Gilberts 'Big Magic' and this gave me the kick start I needed. I imposed a timeline of a year to complete it. I didn't know if I could write a book – did I even have anything to say? Either way I was going to give it my best shot. I got up early most mornings and began to write. Some days were easier than others, but the words started to flow.

Supply teaching was fine and I managed to fit it in around my time with Steven, but I knew I didn't want to be doing it for long. It was just a stop gap. If I went back to full time teaching it meant Steven and I wouldn't be able to see each other as much. I also felt like I'd been there and done that. I wanted something new, something connected with yoga.

As luck would have it I saw an advert for a role of studio co-ordinator at a new yoga studio opening a few miles away. This sounded perfect and I most definitely had the experience. After a long telephone interview I landed a face to face interview. The studio was in the owner's back garden and she asked me to bring answers to a long list of questions. I sat up late preparing. I really wanted this job.

Steven travelled to the interview with me, planning to go to a coffee shop and wait. Instead the owner of the studio saw us together and invited him in to wait in her house. She showed us around the small studio in her garden and although it was nice, it was also clear that she didn't know anything about yoga or running a yoga studio. Steven and I looked at each other realising this had been a complete waste of time. I should have walked out then, but I had prepared hard for this interview, so I wanted to see it through.

The owner was abrupt and had obviously only got me there to pick my brains. She really didn't have a clue and I doubt she even liked yoga. I also realised that she wasn't willing to pay me for the role. I cut the interview short and we went out for lunch.

I shouldn't have raised my hopes, but I was really counting on this job. I believe everything happens for a reason and attending that interview gave me a spark of an idea. I could teach yoga from home!

Although I have a small apartment, the outside decking area is large. If I could get a structure put there then I could offer classes at an affordable price. The more Steven and I talked about it, the more excited I became. There was obviously lots to think about and I didn't know if it would work but I wanted to try.

Yoga For Acceptance

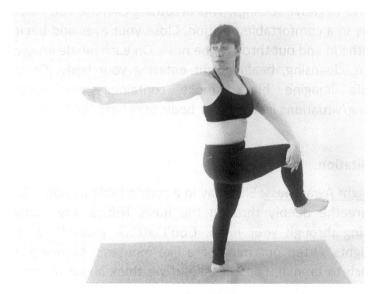

Standing Twist

Pose:

Standing Twist: Begin in a steady standing position (Chapter 8). With your hands on your hips, inhale and lift your right knee so it is in line with your hip (or as close as you can). If you are wobbly, then stay here and breathe steadily. It helps to look at a focus point and press your standing big toe into the ground. To twist, hold your right knee with your left hand. As you twist, gently draw your belly in. Reach your right arm behind you. To test your balance, slowly look over your right shoulder, toward your right fingertips. Stay here for 5 breaths and then repeat on the other side.

Breathing:

Smoke and Light: To accept a situation we often need to release negative feelings. This breathing exercise can help. Sit or lay in a comfortable position. Close your eyes and begin to breathe in and out through the nose. On each inhale imagine a white, cleansing, healing light entering your body. On each exhale imagine black smoke containing any negative feeling/situations leaving your body. Stay here for 2 minutes.

Meditation:

Thought Awareness: Sit or lay in a comfortable position. Begin to breathe deeply through the nose. Notice any thoughts passing through your mind. Don't attach yourself to these thoughts. Often our minds are like monkeys, swinging from branch to branch. For example, if we think about dinner, we then think – I must go shopping – I need to make a list – do I have time to go shopping? – which supermarket is closer? – I shouldn't be thinking about food – I eat too much! And on and on...

In this meditation just notice your thoughts without creating stories around them and without making judgements. Imagine your thoughts are on clouds passing through a blue sky. Begin with practicing this meditation for 2 minutes and gradually begin to stay longer.

Chapter 23: My Own Yoga Studio

I had planned to stay at my job at Studio 666 until the end of my operations. I didn't think I could cope with any change but now I had no choice. Supply teaching was giving me an income but this could only be temporary.

I realised I was holding onto a lot of hurt about how my job at Studio 666 had ended. It had been a huge part of my life for several years so it was very strange. During this time, I also felt negative feelings towards my soon to be sister-in-law. She had questioned why Steven and I wanted to get married. She tried to change our wedding plans to suit her and had made a fuss about paying to come to our wedding.

This drama resulted in Steven breaking out in chronic eczema and I was physically sick. I knew I couldn't let this negativity get to me, so with the help of the practices at the end of this chapter, I began to feel stronger and forgive those people who had wronged me.

I also threw myself into the idea of having my own studio. I'd always wanted to offer low cost yoga – most classes in my area were £12-18, too much for most people. I think everyone should be able to do a weekly class for a reasonable cost.

By now it was the end of April 2017 and with summer fast approaching, I knew I needed to set up quickly. My plan was to get a custom-made heavy duty gazebo on my deck which needed to be extended. I had no idea if people would want to do yoga in a gazebo, but I was willing to use the rest of my savings to find out.

I wrote a business plan and set to work. Once the deck was extended and the gazebo sourced, I ordered enough equipment for 8 students. It wouldn't be the most spacious of studios but I hoped it could work. My garden is very pretty, so I knew that practicing yoga in nature would be a perfect mix.

Once I'd set my mind to it, things began to move quickly. Doing supply as well as trying to juggle everything was difficult but I enjoyed being busy. It took my mind off the constant pain which was beginning to take over my left side. I couldn't wait to have the operation. I hoped it wouldn't be long now.

I planned to open the studio at the end of May 2017. I began to advertise by leafleting the local area, social media and anything else I could think of doing. I threw my heart and soul into this project and it felt good to do something for me. I was sick of working for someone else. It was my time now.

I'd had a feeling last New Year's Eve that there would be a big change in my work life. This was being realised now. I had an excited buzzing in the pit of my tummy and it was great to have something all-consuming to focus on.

Of course I worried that nobody would turn up to the classes. There is a lot of yoga in my area and some great studios. Mine was something completely different, smaller and friendlier and starting at only £6 per class, maybe people would come and give it a try.

On the evening of 31st May 2017, as I opened the side gate to my garden, I hoped at least some people would turn up. It was still a beautiful, hot day which may inspire people to come to class in a garden environment. I'd had some bookings, but as I was taking payment on arrival, I wasn't sure they would show up.

For my first class I had 10 students. My studio only holds 8! Some people thought they could turn up without booking, but thankfully I managed to squeeze them all in. I had 6 students in the second class that night. I was thrilled! They all rebooked for the following week.

During the next few weeks I made steady progress. I had to tweak the timetable a few times and I did have occasions where I only had one student for a class, but on the whole I was getting busier and busier.

The feedback I received was amazing. The students seemed to enjoy my style of teaching and they loved the garden environment. In the warm weather I could open the sides of the gazebo and be surrounded by nature. I enjoyed running my own little studio. Having been repressed at Studio 666 for so long, it was liberating to have my own space and be my own boss.

Over the summer my new business grew and grew. I began teaching 10 classes a week and introduced a programme of workshops as well. I frequently had to turn students away as I was fully booked.

The students who came to my classes were from all walks of life – builders, cleaners, nurses, teachers, actors – many of whom had never thought of doing yoga. They found the large studios too intimidating and costly. My studio was welcoming, reasonably priced, only held small groups and was not pretentious. I knew everyone by name and enjoyed hearing about their lives. Many students told me they saw my studio as 'their sanctuary'.

At the end of the summer, I held a party for the students. As I sat in the fading summer sunshine, I couldn't believe what I had achieved. I had a business that I loved and it was all from my own efforts (and also help, support and guidance from my parents and Steven).

I was surprised and humbled by my success, but I did worry about the winter months. Could I manage to make the gazebo warm enough so the students would stay with me?

I knew I had to choose my wedding dress before my surgery as I wouldn't be mobile enough afterwards. It was difficult to select a dress without knowing exactly how I would look after my next operation. After a disastrous first appointment where I looked old and fat in everything I tried on, in the second appointment I found my perfect dress. It was lightweight, floaty and very pretty. The ideal dress for a cruise ship wedding. I couldn't wait!

My final operation was scheduled for 13th September 2017. I felt I could finally see the light at the end of the tunnel.

Yoga For Letting Go

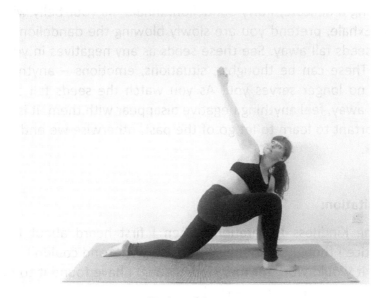

Twisted Lunge

Pose:

<u>Twisted Lunge</u>: Step your right foot forward into a lunge position (Chapter 18). Stay here for a few breaths and gradually move your left knee further back to increase the stretch. Keep your left hand on the mat and place your right hand on your hip. Begin to turn your right shoulder towards the ceiling. As you do this gently draw your belly in to increase the twist. If this feels comfortable, then reach your right arm towards the ceiling. If it hurts your neck to look up, then look towards the floor. Try to keep your right knee drawn to the centre. Encourage your left shoulder away from your ear. Stay here for 5 breaths and then repeat on the other side.

Breathing:

Dandelion Breath: With your hand in front of you, imagine holding a delicate, fluffy dandelion. Inhale, fill your belly with air. Exhale, pretend you are slowly blowing the dandelion so the seeds fall away. See these seeds as any negatives in your life. These can be thoughts, situations, emotions – anything that no longer serves you. As you watch the seeds fall and float away, feel anything negative disappear with them. It is so important to learn to let go of the past, otherwise we end up stuck.

Meditation:

Loving Kindness Meditation: When I first heard about this practice I thought it sounded a bit 'new age' and couldn't see how it would work for me. I was wrong. I have found it to be powerful – so be open minded!

- Sit or lay in a comfortable position and take steady breaths through the nose.

- *Focus on Self*: To begin, send loving energy to yourself by repeating the phrase, 'May I be happy and peaceful, may my body and mind be healthy and strong, may I be safe and protected, may I live with ease and joy.'

- *Someone You Love:* Now think of someone you love very much. Feel their presence around you. Think of the reasons why you love them. Then repeat the same phrase to that person, 'May you be happy and peaceful, may your body and mind be healthy and strong, may you be safe and protected, may you live with ease and joy'.

- *An Acquaintance*: Think of an acquaintance or someone you know but not very well. Think of something you appreciate about that person. Repeat the phrase to that person.

- *Hurt/Dislike*: This is the tricky part! Think of someone who has hurt you, or someone who you do not particularly like. Think of one positive quality of that person if you can. Then repeat the same phrase to that person. It is very natural to find this difficult but just do your best.

- *For Everyone*: To end the meditation, repeat the phrase for everyone in your meditation.

Chapter 24: Rock Bottom

By the beginning of August 2017, I was busy preparing for my final operation. I had found yoga teachers to cover my classes and I'd even booked my usual pre-op eyelash tint. The last thing to do was to stop taking my HRT in a few days' time. The hospital had advised me to stop taking it 4 weeks before surgery as it can increase the risk of blood clots.

The weather was hot and I was going to have a few days away with my Mum for her birthday. We were looking forward to relaxing and lounging around in a spa hotel. On the day we left I received a letter to say my operation had been postponed until 15th November 2017.

I was in constant pain and the temporary implant was very uncomfortable. I quickly phoned the admissions department and explained my situation. I was told that my surgeon had a lot of cancer patients and that's why I had to be bumped from the list. They would make a note on my file not to cancel me again.

I totally understood that cancer patients were priority, but the situation was impacting on my daily life. Steven kept telling me to take painkillers but I didn't want to. I rarely take them anyway and I definitely didn't want to live on them. How could I really move on with my life until after this operation was complete?

My parents, Steven and I were planning a special holiday to celebrate the end of my operations, my parent's 50th wedding anniversary and my 40th birthday which was at the end of the year. But we had to put our plans on hold. We couldn't book anything until I'd had this operation.

Although I was very disappointed the date had been changed, going to the spa hotel soon lifted my spirits. I knew I could handle the pain until November 2017.

Steven and I had organised our work, so we would have a week off for the operation. Rather than waste the week, we decided to go on holiday. Soon we were basking in the sunshine on Lanzarote. The break did me the world of good and the disappointment of the postponed operation did not seem so bad.

On my return, I knew I needed to keep myself busy and healthy for the next two months to prepare for the surgery. I had an earache before the holiday, but it had got worse on the plane and after swimming in the sea. I finally went to the doctor and it turned out I had an ear infection. I'd never had one before. Of course, it was also on my left side (the same side as my temporary implant). It affected my balance so teaching yoga was interesting!

The ear infection was persistent. I went through an antibiotic ear spray and two courses of antibiotics to clear it up. In fact, the whole of my left side felt broken and weak. It was even noticeable in my hair – the left side was shorter than the right and far more damaged. I continued with daily exercise and yoga as I wanted to stay active. My body was crying out for help.

My favourite thing to do during that time was curling up in bed with my book. Usually my cat, Truffles, slept on my feet at the same time. I just really felt I needed the escapism that reading provides. Outwardly I was fine, but inwardly I was tired. So tired of waiting.

The studio was still busy. By the middle of October 2017 we had endured wet, windy and cold weather and the studio was still warm and dry. Steven and I had installed 2 patio heaters near the roof and sprinkled fairy lights throughout. It looked like a winter wonderland.

With four weeks to go before my operation, I stopped taking the HRT. As the date loomed, my fear of receiving a cancellation letter increased. I developed a deep hatred of thin white envelopes. I had a gut feeling the operation would be cancelled. Unfortunately, two and a half weeks before surgery I was proved right. It was moved to the end of February 2018.

I struggled to breathe. February? I couldn't wait until February! I'd waited long enough. I phoned the admissions officer and she told me that Mr H was primarily dealing with cancer patients. The same thing could happen to me in February.

I told her how much pain I was experiencing and explained that this was really impacting on my life. She told me that it may be possible for another surgeon to perform the operation. She would be able to tell me the following week as she would need to present my case in a meeting.

I cried. A lot. I felt hopeless. I also felt very let down by Mr H. I knew he had hundreds of other patients, but I was sure he would want to finish the job he'd started. My parents very kindly said they would pay for the operation to be done privately by Mr H. Initially I refused but when after a week I couldn't get any joy from the NHS I scheduled a private telephone consultation with him for the following week. He was on holiday until then.

My rib cage locked and I had couldn't breathe properly. I think it was the shock. My healer released this area so at least I was a bit more comfortable.

By then I had been off the HRT for two weeks and the effects started to become apparent. I often felt hot as though my blood was boiling and I ached all over. I felt so tired and very teary. I tried to soldier on the best I could. The only things that helped were exercise and yoga. This wasn't always easy due to my extreme pain, but I persevered.

I hit rock bottom the following week. I burst into tears at the drop of a hat, all my energy had ebbed away. I felt sick, dizzy and I lost my appetite. I struggled to get out of bed and I didn't want to see anyone. My short-term memory was compromised and I felt delicate and fragile. I'm not sure how I managed to put on a brave face and teach. I struggled to remember the names of the poses and I had to swallow back my tears. It was miserable. I was miserable.

My parents and Steven did their best to support me but nobody really knew what to do. It was very cruel – my body was screaming for the oestrogen it was lacking so I would feel normal again. I was also dealing with the uncertainty of my surgery date. I didn't want to start taking HRT again in case I did get a slot for my operation in the coming weeks.

My life was once again on hold. Steven and I couldn't book train tickets to see each other as the surgery could be anytime. My Dad and I regularly go to The Royal Opera House but booking tickets was out of the question. I was very, very frustrated.

It took a few weeks for my body to regulate. I still felt as though I was lacking something, but the tears had dried up and I felt better. Teaching became easier but I was still physically and mentally drained. I felt as though I was being tortured from within. I was in so much pain.

Following the telephone consultation with Mr H he scheduled my operation privately in January 2018. He had very kindly offered to try to get me moved forward on the NHS list, but I knew I would probably be cancelled yet again. I had to get this over with. Even though we were going private I would still have two months to wait.

I felt angry and miserable. The reason for this intense pain was that the implant had been overinflated and moved in front of the muscle. It was probably pressing on a nerve. It felt as though I was dragging my left side around with me each day.

I had a decision to make – I could spend the next two months being miserable or I could make the best of things. I chose the latter. I organised a charity event at my studio and raised £500 for Crisis at Christmas. I also held a festive party which was packed out and a big success. I just took it one day at a time and accepted my temporary pain.

Steven took me away for my 40th birthday to a beautiful hotel. We had a fantastic time but by this time, the end of 2017, the shooting pains down my left side were horrendous. I knew I only had 2 weeks to go until my operation and I was counting the days. I rarely slept as the pain was so bad. I was exhausted.

Yoga For Anger

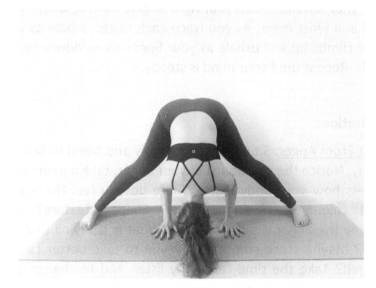

Wide Legged Forward Fold

Pose:

<u>Wide Legged Forward Fold</u>: Step your feet wider than your shoulders, your toes should be pointing forward. Bend your knees and bring your hands to your hips. Inhale, lift your chest and exhale, fold your torso forward. Make sure you fold at your hips and do not round your lower back. Place your hands on the floor or blocks so they are shoulder distance apart. Bring your weight forward on to the balls of your feet. Draw your belly up and in and gently lengthen your chest towards the floor. Roll your shoulders away from your ears and draw your shoulder blades together. Relax your head. If it feels comfortable then straighten your legs. Stay here for 5-10 breaths. To come out of the pose, bend your knees, place your hands on your hips and roll up to standing.

Breathing:

Finger Breathing: Sit comfortably with a straight spine. Slowly trace your left hand with your right finger, starting where your hand and wrist meet. As you trace each finger, inhale as your finger climbs up and exhale as your finger slides down. Switch hands. Repeat until your mind is steady.

Meditation:

A Gift From Anger: Sit or lay comfortably and begin to breathe deeply. Notice the sensations of your anger, take a moment to witness how your body feels. Where do you feel the anger? What colour is it? Temperature? Shape? Texture? Now imagine the anger is a good friend. What is it saying that you need? Maybe stuck emotions? Maybe to take better care of yourself? Take the time to quietly listen and to change your relationship with anger. Remember all emotions are natural and we can learn from each one.

Chapter 25: Looking Ahead

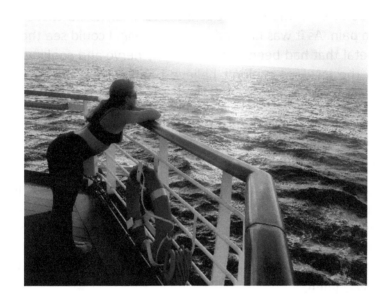

The great thing about having a private operation is it's unlikely to be cancelled. You also have more pleasant surroundings and your own room. When my operation date, 9th January 2018, finally come around I felt as though I had checked into a hotel.

There was no waiting in hot corridors, no carrying your own pillow and no hospital smell. It was like a dream. I wasn't at all nervous, just so eager to be operated on. I had waited for this day for over a year. As they anaesthetised me, I didn't care how I ended up looking, I just wanted the pain to go away.

Before I knew it, I was being wheeled back from surgery to my own room where my parents and Steven were waiting. Even though I was groggy and sore on my left side, I could instantly feel that the shooting pains had gone. It was such a relief. As I sat in my room eating smoked salmon finger sandwiches (what a cliché!) I felt elated.

I chose to keep the implant as a souvenir as it had caused so much pain. As it was handed to me in a bag, I could see the bit of metal that had been pressing on my nerve and cooking me from the inside. I couldn't believe I had carried this around with me for 15 months.

I gave myself a week off from the studio and began the healing process that I'd been through so many times. Now it was different. Hopefully this was the end.

I'd got to the point where I couldn't remember what it felt like to be 'normal'. I was so used to being in pain all the time and so used to feeling exhausted due to lack of oestrogen. I could finally begin taking the HRT my body needed. It took a few weeks, but my energy began to return and the pain in my left side was gone.

During my check-up appointment with Mr H he told me he couldn't believe how well the reconstruction had turned out. He said that when they inserted the temporary implant during my second breast operation, he didn't hold out much hope for me keeping the breast. I knew I had come close to losing it but hearing him say this made me realise I am so lucky.

Just as I was getting my strength back and beginning to teach again I had dreadful problems with my studio. I had leak after leak during a particularly cold, snowy and windy February 2018.

The gazebo had weathered well up to this point. My Dad, Steven and I worked for hours in the freezing cold to try and fix things. At one point it looked like I would have to close the studio. The floor was pulled up and re-laid more times than I can remember. New side panels were added. Clearing snow from the top of the gazebo and the long entrance path became the norm.

My gazebo seems to have a mind and spirit of its own. There's often no particular reason why it leaks, has condensation or holds in heat. It's like teaching with a partner who is very unpredictable. It does however have a special inner energy which people sense. Combined with a lovely garden environment, it makes it a very special place to practice yoga.

Just after this, Steven, my parents and I managed to escape the wintery weather and go on our greatly anticipated holiday. We had an amazing 2 weeks cruising around the Caribbean. The relaxed atmosphere and hot sunshine restored us and it was lovely to spend time together.

I returned with new energy, teaching in a more creative way. Ideas for classes seemed to flow and my body felt better than it had in years. I lost the stubborn half a stone I had put on during all the trauma and my strength continued to grow. I also finally got around to finishing this book!

So how do I feel now?

I feel I have survived just as my studio has survived. A bit weather beaten and with new parts but still essentially the same.

My body and mind continue to heal; I know this will take many years. I need to show myself kindness and patience.

Of course I have scars but overall I'm pleased with my body. In clothes you can't tell that I've had a breast reconstruction (in fact the photos in this book were taken post surgeries) and I do have a lot of sensation back.

My new favourite pastime is shopping for bras. After over a year and a half in a sports bra, it's very liberating. The scars on my tummy are barely visible. I'm not sure why but I have thicker hair and better skin than before.

I'm relieved that I've zoomed through the menopause and I don't have that looming over me in the coming years. I still feel just as feminine and I don't have any menopausal symptoms.

The relief of stepping off the treadmill of hospital appointments is immense. I can finally make plans and get on with my life. The yearly check ups will always be there, but for the most part, my traumatic time can begin to fade into the background.

As a Reiki healer I now feel energy flow much more strongly through my left hand. My left side had all the problems so I'm not sure why this is the case, but I know I am a more powerful healer now.

There is a risk I could have gone through all of this and still end up with cancer as it's impossible to remove all the tissue. I still look out for signs of breast and ovarian cancer, but I don't let this rule my life.

There have been many times I wished I didn't know about my gene mutation. Ignorance can be bliss. But more importantly, knowledge is power. I know I have done everything in my ability to be able to live a long and healthy life. I find this comforting.

In hindsight, I realise that all my past experiences had prepared me to be able to go through this process. From having a positive mind set to becoming a yoga teacher. I was lucky to have the right tools to help myself heal.

I feel resilient and ready for any more challenges that life will, I'm sure, throw at me. I allow life to flow through me. My studio is going from strength to strength and I'm teaching with passion. Working outside in nature continues to heal me day by day.

In 2 months I'm getting married and I can't wait! I'm ready for the next chapter of my life.

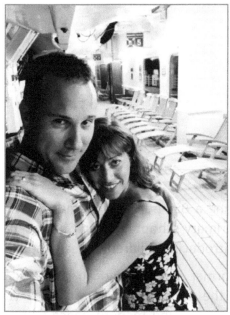

Steven & Me

About Sarah

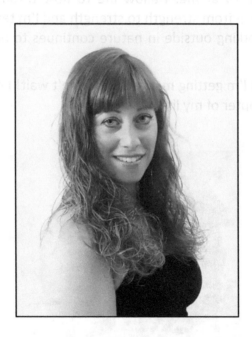

After completing a BSc honours degree in psychology, Sarah trained as a primary school teacher. She taught for 12 years and enjoyed introducing children to health and fitness.

Sarah is a former Latin American and Ballroom dancer, competing in the UK and abroad for many years. She also trained in ballet, tap and modern dance when she attended The BRIT Performing Arts and Technology School.

Sarah has been in the fitness industry for over 10 years. She is a qualified Zumba, spin and boxing teacher as well as a personal trainer. She strives to make all her classes fun and energising.

Sarah discovered yoga 15 years ago. She loved the feeling of her body gently opening up and found that the meditative effects had a positive impact on her well-being. She was able to think more clearly, had less injuries and more energy. Sarah then wanted to pass these benefits on to others.

Initially travelling to Mexico to attend an intensive yoga teacher training programme, she has since immersed herself in other trainings. These include Hot Power Yoga, Yin Yoga, Forrest Yoga and she is a qualified Reiki healer.

Sarah teaches Vinyasa Flow, Power and Yin/Restorative Yoga. She focuses on alignment and allowing people to find the safest expression of their movements. She enjoys using her knowledge of dance to sequence postures in a creative way. Her guidance is clear, heartfelt and she enjoys sharing her love of yoga with others.

She became tired of the large, impersonal yoga studios that dominate and prefers to teach small groups, therefore giving each student more attention. Sarah also does not agree with the high cost of most yoga classes as she believes that yoga should be available to everyone. This has led her to create a unique yoga studio 'Sarah Brown Yoga @The Cabin'. A sanctuary where everyone can come for classes at a reasonable price.

Sarah decided to write this book to chronicle her experiences of learning she carried the BRCA gene mutation and going through the ordeal of risk reducing surgery.

www.sarahbrownyoga.co.uk

info@sarahbrownyoga.co.uk